Microwave Cooking for Your Baby and Child

The Pregnancy Diet

*Fit Kids: Raising Physically and Emotionally
Strong Kids with Real Food*

Meals That Heal for Babies, Toddlers, and Children

Therapeutic Nutrition: A Guide to Patient Education

Cooking Well for the Unwell

*Eat Well, Lose Weight, While Breastfeeding:
The Complete Nutrition Book for Nursing Mothers*

THE BABY FOOD BIBLE

THE BABY FOOD BIBLE

A Complete Guide
to Feeding Your
Child, from
Infancy On

EILEEN BEHAN

BALLANTINE BOOKS NEW YORK

A Ballantine Books Trade Paperback Original

Copyright © 2008 by Eileen Behan

All rights reserved.

Published in the United States by Ballantine Books, an imprint of The Random House Publishing Group, a division of Random House, Inc., New York.

BALLANTINE and colophon are registered trademarks of Random House, Inc.

Library of Congress Cataloging-in-Publication Data
Behan, Eileen.
The baby food bible : a complete guide to feeding your child, from infancy on / Eileen Behan.
p.   cm.
Includes bibliographical references and index.
ISBN 978-0-345-50085-4 (pbk.)
1. Infants—Nutrition—Popular works.
2. Toddlers—Nutrition—Popular works.   I. Title.

RJ216.B338   2008
649'.3—dc22
2008006177

Printed in the United States of America

www.ballantinebooks.com

8 9

Book design by Jo Anne Metsch

To my parents,
John and Elizabeth Behan;
thank you for everything

Acknowledgments

Special gratitude goes to my family—Sheila, Kevin, and Agi; my husband, David; and daughters Sarah and Emily—who are always willing and honest participants in the sharing of ideas, theories, and meals. I would like to thank the extended McCue family for always asking, "So, what are you working on now?" and being encouraging about what I tell them.

This book would not have been possible without the medical and health specialists who research and publish about pediatric nutrition. Their work is credited in the back of these pages; without their data and statistics all I would have to say would be just commentary and opinion. In particular, I would like to thank Kathleen C. Bloomer ARNP for reading the manuscript cover to cover for accuracy on medical issues. A very special thanks to Jane Hackett MA, RD, CDE, LD for her review of nutrition content and the addition of ideas. To Judith Paige RD, Marilyn DeSimone RD, and Madeleine Walsh RD a very special thanks for all their contributions and support.

This book is in large part inspired by the individuals I have worked with at Core Services, whose questions about food, nutrition, and diet made me see the need for this book, and the staff and providers, who give me the opportunity to make a difference in their patients' lives.

Thanks to Trish Cronan and Brad Lavigne, who are always enthusiastic and interested in my work, and to Conni White and Lisa Connors for their goodwill and humor.

A special thanks to Megan Ross, Lisa Kumph, Dawn Sciascia, Christina Couperthwait, Alison Petersen, Kathleen Beede, Elizabeth Winter, Sharon McGovern, and Carla Snow—parents who made this a better book by sharing their insights, successes, and concerns about feeding their children.

A huge thanks goes to Kate Cunningham Wilker for reading and commenting on whatever and however much I sent her while raising Graham and Oliver.

To my agent, Carol Mann, for finding a good home for this book. I would like to thank my editor Rebecca Shapiro, and the others at Random House, including Nancy Delia and Robbin Schiff.

Contents

Introduction . . . . *xiii*

ONE This Is Not Your Mother's Kitchen. *3*

TWO The Easy Year. *9*

THREE Feeding Your Toddler *36*

FOUR Superior Foods. *52*

FIVE High Chair Cuisine. *113*

SIX The Family Table *136*

SEVEN How to Shop *184*

EIGHT How to Raise a Healthy Eater *192*

NINE Effective Parenting. *202*

TEN Feeding Your Preschooler. *207*

ELEVEN Confusing Issues. *214*

References *237*

Index. *243*

Introduction

Your baby depends on you for everything. You will make sure she is safe and warm, you will do your best to anticipate her needs, and you will try to determine what is wrong when she cries. You will give great thought to every decision you make about your child's well-being, and you will ask questions when you need information. Nutrition is no different. Very quickly your child will move from breast milk or formula to baby food and then on to table food. You will give considerable attention to what she eats and how you prepare it, but unlike previous generations who lived with real concerns about food scarcity and malnutrition, you live in a world of unprecedented food abundance. With that comes unique parenting concerns that no other generation of parents has had to face.

Today a thousand new food items are introduced each month. Young children watch more than eight thousand television commercials each year telling them what to eat. That means that the favorite vegetable of two-year-old children is french fries, and cola sodas are becoming the breakfast beverage of choice. Heart disease accounts for 30 percent of deaths around the world; high blood pressure affects more than 25 percent of adults and is on the rise in children. Rates of obesity among children have tripled in the past three decades. Concurrently, type 2 diabetes has become an epidemic; the prevalence of diagnosis in the United States has increased by 61 percent in the past decade alone. Billions of dollars have been spent on public health projects to educate school-age children in an attempt to reverse the trend in diet-related diseases. None of these programs has been very effective. Unless we take a new approach, it is almost certain that more and more of our children will be impacted, and for the first time your child's generation may not live longer than the previous generation.

Obesity is never an issue in infancy. The environment that creates obesity later on, however, is very much a parenting issue. You can protect your child against the obesity epidemic and its diet-related illnesses by taking an approach to eating and feeding that replaces the current food environment with one that promotes optimal health and strong family relations. Two simple principles will allow you to be successful at this: establish and protect family mealtime, and introduce your child to a variety of truly good food. Your goal is to create an environment that allows your child to develop his natural feeding abilities, and you can do that by serving predictable meals that include a variety of foods, choosing snacks thoughtfully, and eating as a family as often as you can. In this book I will try to answer all nutrition questions with the most accurate and current information available, to help you be a confident parent prepared to guide your child through a complicated food world.

As I write this book my daughters are now eighteen and twenty years old, and I am proud that they have developed good eating habits beyond noodles and apples, which is all they seemed to want as children. When they were young I worried about their desire for sweets, their limited interest in vegetables, and their preference for fruit over vegetables. I watched what they ate, and I had to work hard to avoid interfering with their natural ability to self-regulate. One daughter was a robust eater and the other a dabbler. As a parent, I did the best I could. With the intention of raising healthy kids, I learned about food, I served good food, and I created family meals as a part of that effort. I believe food and family meals are a way to develop rituals that create security. Meals can be an expression of caring and love.

For the past twenty years I have been a practicing nutritionist, talking with thousands of parents about food and family. I know with certainty that the way parents feed their children in the first twenty-four months will lay the foundation for their future health. I also know that right now, as you develop your ideas about parenting and strive to make the best decisions for your baby, is the time to reach you and influence your food and meal choices.

For some of you, cooking and meal preparation can be a source of stress—perhaps because you think you are not good at it, you worry about poor food choices, or you fear that if you enjoy food too much it could cause disordered eating in your child when she becomes older. Many of you have struggled with your own food issues; combine this with the news that diet-related disease, obesity, and eating disorders are on the rise and it can make any parent anxious. There are very real and serious issues related to diet. But if you want to create a healthy attitude regarding food, you can't be afraid to use good food as your ally. I believe enjoying food is a way to prevent future food issues.

In Chapter 1, "This Is Not Your Mother's Kitchen," I will describe how the food world has changed over the past thirty years and what that means to you and your family. Chapter 2, "The Easy Year," gets its name because feeding decisions in your child's first year, while new and unfamiliar to you, are not the difficult ones. Chapter 3, "Feeding Your Toddler," provides a month-by-month feeding schedule and describes common feeding problems and what can be done about them. Chapter 4, "Superior Foods," describes more than a hundred foods you will want to include in your baby's and toddler's menu as soon as appropriate. This chapter will also describe inferior foods, the foods that will undermine your efforts to eat well because they replace superior foods. In Chapter 5, "High Chair Cuisine," you will find recipes that meet your child's nutritional and developmental needs in the first eighteen months of life. These recipes are based on what I fed my own girls as well as tips I've received from parents who care about food. I encourage parents to serve from the family table as soon as possible. Chapter 6, "The Family Table," provides recipes that can be prepared for the whole family and then turned into baby food by simply pureeing, mashing, or mixing to meet your baby's needs. In Chapter 7, "How to Shop," I address the food controversies that impact what we buy, such as the ethical treatment of animals, growth hormones in food, organic food, and the importance of country-of-origin labeling. In Chapter 8, "How to Raise a Healthy Eater," readers have a stage-by-stage guide that anticipates the feeding issues that will almost certainly emerge as your child grows and is introduced to new foods, and provides suggestions for coping with them. Chapter 9, "Effective Parenting," describes strategies for positive parenting, including how to use language and modeling behavior to support your goals of good health and a strong family. In Chapter 10, "Feeding Your Preschooler," how and what to feed the three-to-six-year-old child is addressed. For many of you this is a long way off, but for those with older children at home it will give guidance on how to apply the healthy feeding advice for little ones to your older children. Finally, Chapter 11, "Confusing Issues," answers real parent questions on topics such as food allergies, colic, constipation, and much more.

You are your child's most important teacher, and it is up to you to instill in him a desire for good food while protecting him from an environment that tells him to overeat. By taking care of your own child's nutrition and making informed food choices, it is possible to have an impact that transcends your family. Your family's food choices can impact menus at gatherings of your extended family, at school fund-raisers, and even where you work. Nutritionists worry that this generation could have more diet-related diseases and live shorter lives. But it is also possible that this generation could avoid the pitfalls of the previous generation and actually create a world where the trend in diet-related diseases is reversed. My intention is to give you the information to do just that. This book is a resource for the current generation of parents to reverse the trend in diet-related diseases. Please read my ideas and try them on; if they fit for your family, use them and pass them on.

THE BABY FOOD BIBLE

ONE

This Is Not Your Mother's Kitchen

Your food choices are more complex now than at any other time in history. When your great-grandmother went shopping, she had only nine hundred food items to choose from at the local market. Your supermarket, on the other hand, is likely to carry forty-five thousand items. Some additions have been positive, including a greater variety of fruits and vegetables and certainly more whole grains and even organic food. But it is the addition of what I call inferior foods that is alarming. Over the past decade the snack food market has increased by 25 percent, with more than $60 million in sales. The baby food aisle alone contains mini granola bars, ready-to-eat meals, and snack treats. High-fructose corn syrup, an ingredient in almost all of those snack items, was created in 1960; according to an article in the *American Journal of Nutrition,* its use has increased by 1,000 percent per capita—and, I fear, permanently altered young people's desire for sweet-tasting food.

Parents often don't believe me when I say food is cheaper today, but it is. According to the *Nutrition Action Healthletter,* Americans spent, in the 1950s, 21 percent of their disposable income on food, while in the year 2000 only 11 percent of our disposable income was spent on food. Cheaper food means that in order to make money, the American food industry must get us and our children to overeat. The American food industry daily produces 3,900 calories' worth of food for every man, woman, and child in the country, an amount that is almost double what the average adult actually needs and way above what a young child requires.

How we eat has changed, too. The number of meals that families eat together has declined, snacking has replaced real meals, and the microwave has become a part of almost every home. The impact of these changes has been a dramatic increase in childhood obesity, an accompanying rise in disease, and a potentially reduced life span.

You and your child are at risk of poor food choices and the resulting health risks because of advertising, the wide availability of food, and our innate biology. For example, in 2004 Kraft Foods spent $26 million just on advertising the children's deli meat product called Lunchables—a truly inferior food because of its excessive sodium content and lack of vitamins and fiber. Coca-Cola spends $1 billion each year advertising its products. These products (and others like them) are in your child's future. The combination of ubiquitous advertising, wide availability, and low price makes food flavored with salt, sugar, and fat almost impossible for a child (and her parents) to self-limit. In addition to all the societal factors, human beings are simply "wired" to eat them. Our ancestors learned a very long time ago that foods with fat had more calories and would keep them alive, foods with a sweet taste were not likely to be poisonous, and salt—a nutrient essential to health but so hard to find in nature—was to be consumed whenever available. All human beings—including you and your child—are physiologically designed to covet these tastes.

The food world in which you are raising your child is different because of all these products, but also because the American family eats away from home more often. On any given night only 58 percent of us are eating at home, and many of those meals include take-out restaurant food or store-bought convenience products. Pizza, burgers, and Chinese are the most popular take-out foods, and they will soon be part of your child's diet, too.

You might think that the world I describe above does not yet apply to your baby; babies are perceived to live in this rarefied bubble that protects them from the world of adult concerns. Say the words "baby food" and you are likely to picture tiny bowls of smooth warm oatmeal and creamy orange carrots. Those images may be accurate for some babies, but not for all. There is a discrepancy between what babies need to eat and what babies actually are being fed. Half of all seven-to-eight-month-olds are eating dessert daily; the dessert replaces the recommended fruits and vegetables they actually need. One-third of seven-to-twenty-four-month-old babies eat no vegetables at all, and by fifteen months french fries become the most popular vegetable.

The Feeding Infants and Toddler Study (FITS), published in 2004, was a study sponsored by the Gerber Products Company to update our understanding of the food and nutrient intakes of infants and toddlers in the United States. The survey asked parents or caregivers about the feeding habits of their children age four months to twenty-four months. It gives us a look into what real families are feeding their kids and is useful because it illustrates how quickly parents are forced to make decisions about how and what they feed their child. The survey also covered food choices, feeding practices, growth and development, and nutrient intake. The results were mixed.

The FITS data suggest that most babies have been introduced to solid foods by four to six months. At this early age children are just learning to eat and become familiar with food, so a "balanced diet" isn't an issue since formula and breast milk are the true nutritional safety net. The majority of babies have had some sort of grain product (usually infant cereal) by six months, and about 40 percent are eating a little fruit and vegetable. Less than 1 percent have had a dessert or sweetened beverage. By eleven months, the majority of babies (98 percent) are eating grains (cereal, bread), and over 70 percent have fruits, vegetables, and meats in their menu. Few infants are getting plain meats; instead, parents are opting for baby food combination dinners. Few children are eating the recommended servings of dark green vegetables, and once they move to table food, potatoes become the vegetable of choice. Eleven percent of eleven-month-olds have been served soda or fruit-flavored drinks, and by twenty-four months the proportion of babies consuming sweetened beverages jumps to 44 percent, 60 percent eat a baked dessert, and 20 percent get candy.

Children given more sweetened drinks early in life are likely to consume more sweet drinks later. Sweetened drinks are so easy to consume in excess, crowding out other more nutritious foods, that the American Academy of Pediatrics (AAP) now recommends only 6 ounces of 100 percent fruit juice per day and no fruit drinks or soda. Apple juice and apple-flavored fruit drinks are popular baby beverages, and for many children fruit drinks and soda replace milk by age two. At this age some infants are drinking little or no milk, possibly leading to low calcium intake if non-milk sources are not consumed as alternatives.

The FITS survey shows that the trend of not meeting the recommendations for fruit and vegetables starts as early as nine to eleven months. As babies transition to table food, 25 percent of nineteen-to-twenty-four-month-olds are consuming chips or other salty snacks on any given day. This is significant because the foods introduced in the early years can impact a child's preference for life. These trends make it important for you to examine your own eating and drinking habits. Your child will want to eat what you are eating, and if Mom and Dad are having french fries and sweetened drinks, most babies will, too.

The rise in childhood obesity should be no surprise, as it mirrors adult issues. Those in the lower socioeconomic brackets are hit the hardest. The rate of obesity for middle- and high-income American adults is 29 percent, but the rate for low-income Americans is 35 percent, and low-income kids have a similarly high percentage of being overweight. Overweight in adults is defined as having a Body Mass Index (BMI) between 25 and 30. Over 30 is considered obese. In children a BMI above the ninety-fifth percentile for the child's age is considered overweight.

Combine the fact that adults have complex food choices with the phenomenon of the "picky eater" and you have a source of real stress for new parents. As many as 50 percent of babies four to twenty-four months of age are described by their parents as picky eaters. A picky eater can grow up in any family, and it is not an indicator of good or bad parenting. It is so common it must be normal. That doesn't mean nothing can be done to prevent it. Most parents offer a food three to five times before deciding their child does not like it, but that may not be enough—children may need eight to fifteen tries before accepting a food. Don't give up—the more variety you give your child, the more you may influence the flavors and textures he actually accepts. Read more about the picky eater on page 46.

The good news is that despite the introduction of dessert, sweetened beverages, and salty snacks, children are not deficient in nutrients. Surveys consistently show adequate intake of nutrients, in part due to the fortification of foods. That is not the same as saying babies and children are eating well, because the bad news is they are not eating enough fruit, vegetables, and good calcium choices—foods containing unique substances that prevent illness and promote good health. Not eating sufficient amounts from the recommended food groups is significant because poor nutrition contributes to high blood pressure, diabetes, heart disease, and obesity—disease processes that all begin in youth.

I am not trying to scare you, but I do want to impress on you that the food you choose really matters. You have to be your child's advocate because your baby is growing up in a food world that many nutritionists describe as "toxic."

The news about food is not all gloomy. Most Americans eat a home-cooked meal almost five times per week, and while fruit and vegetable consumption is not where it should be, the latest food surveys find fresh fruit consumption is on the rise, particularly in families with young children. Concerns about health affect food choices. Parents look for foods described as healthy, "light," and even organic. More than 70 percent of you are breastfeeding your baby for at least part of the first year because you know it is the best way to feed your infant. If we encourage these trends, we'll be off to a much better, healthier start.

HOW TO START OFF RIGHT

Children do not need to be taught how much to eat, but you must support this by showing them how to recognize feelings of hunger and satiety and by feeding them when hungry and allowing them to stop eating when they indicate a sense of fullness. Never force or bribe a child to eat. You do need to choose good food for children because they can't do that on their own.

Babies never need a low-fat or reduced-calorie diet. In the first year of life adult feeding guidelines that encourage low-fat choices do not apply to infants. But that is not the same as saying babies need a menu of high-fat foods.

As soon as you start feeding your baby solid food, you will be forced to make decisions that can affect your child's future health. These food choices are not trivial. Between 75 and 95 percent of major chronic disease is linked to poor nutrition. Good nutrition and activity can prevent chronic illness, and feeding exposures early in life can make a difference. I want to reassure you that selecting food is not complex. It means getting back to basics, recognizing that food choices matter, and knowing how to distinguish the good from the bad.

The Easy Year

Given all the changes that a baby brings to a parent's life, you might be surprised to hear me refer to your child's first year of life as the "easy year." But when it comes to food, the first twelve months really are easy. In the beginning the only feeding choice you make is whether to breastfeed or give formula, and if you are reading this book at home with your newborn by your side, that decision has already been made. Your next decision will be when to add solids and which foods to choose. If you stick to traditional baby food items, either homemade or jarred, the choices are not too complex, either, at least in the beginning. But new parents worry about a lot of things. When I brought my babies home I worried about what it meant when they cried, and I worried about when to start real food and if they were getting enough to eat. The truth is there are no hard-and-fast rules. Breastfed babies should be offered the breast on demand—as much as ten to twelve times a day in the first month; settling into five to ten times per day later on—and in the first few months a baby on formula can drink 18 to 32 ounces divided into four to eight feedings.

It is in these early days that you will want to learn to trust your child's innate ability to self-regulate and know how much he or she needs to eat. Your job is to provide the food in a relaxed and secure environment; if you feed your baby on demand, she will consume exactly the amount she needs. In this early phase I think breastfeeding moms have it easier because they can't see their breast empty of milk in the same way a parent can see a formula bottle empty. Parents feeding with a bottle may think it is their responsibility to teach a child to finish the bottle, but the real job is to allow the child to take what she needs and only finish the bottle if her hunger tells her to do so. The child who falls asleep, refuses the nipple, or stops sucking is indicating that she is no longer hungry. Now is the time to practice trusting your child to consume enough food based on what she needs and not on the amount that fits into a bottle. It is the same skill your child will need when she begins eating from a plate.

CRYING

Please don't let well-meaning friends or family members discourage you from responding to your baby when he cries. Crying is an effective way for a baby to communicate hunger and discomfort, and I believe strongly that the parent who responds to a crying child with a change of diaper, a warm blanket, food, or a gentle cuddle is absolutely not creating a spoiled child but is instead helping the child to feel secure, strong, and important. Babies do not cry because they are trying to manipulate; they cry because they can't talk. You will learn very soon to distinguish a hunger cry from a sick cry, a scared cry, or a pained cry, and you will know what to do. As your baby gets older, routines and a flexible schedule regarding feeding and naps and diaper changes will help you and your baby create a family rhythm that makes you more confident and the baby more secure.

KNOWING WHEN YOUR BABY IS READY FOR SOLID FOOD

Breast milk and formula can meet a baby's nutrient needs through six months and even longer, but many babies are developmentally ready to start solid foods as early as four to six months. It will be important for your baby to move to solid foods to meet her needs for nutrients such as iron, zinc, and vitamin D. While many parents introduce foods earlier than a baby might actually need them, you don't want to wait too long, either. Breastfeeding moms may want to focus on adding solid foods instead of formula, because once formula is introduced it can displace breast milk.

Many parents are ready to start solids early—some because they think the milk feedings are "thin and watery" and believe their child must be hungry for food, others because they think it will help the baby sleep through the night (which does not seem to be true). Some parents believe that adding food to a baby's menu is a developmental milestone. Thirty to 50 percent of babies are given cereal by two to three months of age, and by four to six months 50 to 70 percent of babies are eating cereal. Infant cereal fortified with iron is a common first food because it is easy to use and well tolerated. Additionally, cereal is a source of iron, which is a nutrient that children need to obtain from food around that time, as the stores they were born with are used up and need to be replaced. But it is essential that milk feedings remain a part of your child's diet for the entire first year of life because they are the primary source of the nutrients your child needs.

Ask your health care provider about when to add solid foods. Most will suggest you wait until your child can hold his head up and sit independently. A child who can sit forward to show interest in food or turn his head to show disinterest will be able to communicate hunger and fullness.

HOW TO TELL WHEN YOUR BABY IS HUNGRY

An infant can communicate hunger by crying, moving arms and legs in an excited manner, opening her mouth, and, when older, moving toward the spoon as it approaches. A baby who coos, smiles, and stares at her caregiver may be communicating a desire to continue to eat. Some babies will fall asleep when full, eat very slowly, become fussy, spit out food, turn their head, or refuse the spoon when it is offered as a way to show they are full. You will learn your baby's cues for hunger and fullness very quickly. Now is the time to support your child's ability to self-regulate. When she acts disinterested in eating, don't try to force, coerce, or cajole her to eat a little more. Instead, read those cues and stop feeding. Parents who offer three meals a day along with well-timed snacks never need to be worried about underfeeding their child. Read the early meal guidelines in the box on pages 15–16.

EQUIPMENT NEEDED TO START FEEDING SOLIDS

I have never been a big proponent of baby gadgets, but four infant and baby feeding tools are important enough to be called essential. A good sturdy high chair that is strong and easy to clean will make your life easier and your baby's life safer. In the beginning, you can feed your child in an infant seat, but only if it can be locked into a secure position that allows your child to sit upright. By six months the high chair will become the place to feed the baby. The chair should have a tray that slips on and off easily for cleaning, and the legs should be spaced far enough apart so tipping is not a concern. Make sure it has a safety strap, and be sure to use it—don't expect the tray to hold your baby in place.

Second, you will need an assortment of bibs. I like the stiff heavy plastic types that are easy to wipe off, and I like to have a pocket at the bottom because it catches at least some of the food that inevitably falls. A spoon designed for a child's mouth is important; a regular teaspoon is just too big. Most children do not use a cup until around eight months, though of course there are exceptions to this. I like the cups with screw-on lids. In the beginning, choose one with a small air hole, so that the milk comes out slower. Toddlers will want a lidded cup with two or more air holes to make drinking easier. Finally, choose appropriate plates. A plate should be unbreakable, and as your child gets older and uses his hands and plays at the table, you will want the type that has the suction cups attached. The suction cup allows the plate to stay firmly attached to the tray, making it easier for your baby to eat from, and when your child is older it cannot be picked up and tossed.

WATER

Breast milk and formula provide your baby with enough water. An external source of water can fill up a tiny tummy, and if water replaces breast milk or formula, salt levels in the blood could get too low. In very hot or humid climates or if prolonged diarrhea develops, an additional source of water may be needed. Your health care provider will give you guidance if that arises. Otherwise, keep an eye on your baby's diaper, since wet diapers are a good indicator of adequate hydration. If you introduce juice, add it after six months of age, and keep it to only 4–6 ounces per day. Excessive juice consumption can replace more nutritious foods, and too much juice can lead to diarrhea. Read more about water on page 109.

How to Tell When Your Baby May Be Ready for Solid Food

Here are some clues to a child's readiness for solid food.

- He can sit up with assistance.
- His weight has doubled since birth, or he weighs 13 pounds or more.
- He is hungry after his regular nursing sessions (six to eight times per day) or he drinks 32 ounces of formula.

FOODS TO FEED FIRST

There is no evidence that any particular order of introducing food is important, but most parents choose cereal because of convenience and nutrition. Infant cereal fortified with iron and B vitamins can be a good first food. Mixing it with breast milk or formula can enhance acceptance. It is important in the beginning to offer single-ingredient foods and offer new foods one at a time at intervals of two to four days so you can identify if a new food is not well tolerated or causes an allergic reaction. Introduce combination dinners only after you know that the individual ingredients are well tolerated. Introducing your baby to a wide variety of flavors and textures in the first two years of life may increase his willingness to try new foods later on. If you have breastfed your baby, he has probably already experienced changes in flavor based on the foods you have eaten, and this is a good thing because it, too, increases the willingness to try new foods. Many babies need to try a food eight to fifteen times before it becomes familiar and accepted. Too many parents offer food two or three times and if it is refused don't offer it again, limiting the child's food choices before he has even had a chance to learn what he likes.

What is most important is that you continue with breast milk or formula as the primary source of nutrition for the entire first year. The addition of solid food will teach your baby to eat and to become familiar with food, but during the first twelve months it does not replace the milk feeding.

SUCCESSFUL FIRST SOLID MEAL

Pick the right time. Don't try the first feeding of solid food at a time when your baby is crying out for her usual formula or breast milk—things will not go well. Give her the regular feeding, then offer her some solid food, such as infant cereal prepared with formula or breast milk. Make sure she is sitting upright and secure in your lap or a high chair. Use only a small spoon that fits the shape of her mouth. Keep the portions small. She will be curious about food, but she may not like it. Be patient, don't push it, and remember to smile. If your child does not eat solid food, formula or breast milk is her nutritional safety net for almost the entire first year, so relax!

INFANT FEEDING GUIDE

Use the amounts listed as a guide, and ask your child's health care provider for additional help. At around six months, your baby will develop the palmar grasp, the ability to hold food in the palm, followed by the development of the pincer grasp, which allows the

Age	Food	Amounts per Day	Comments
Birth to six months	Breast milk/formula	18–32 ounces first three months 28–45 ounces three to six months	From birth to six months, the milk feeding (either breast milk or infant formula) is the most important source of nutrition.
Four to six months	Infant cereal Breast milk/formula	4–8 tablespoons 28–45 ounces	After four months many babies are developmentally able to try solid foods, but breast milk and infant formula are much richer in protein than cereal and continue to be the most important food.
Six to eight months	Plain fruit, strained	3–4 tablespoons	At six to eight months, add strained vegetables and fruits and ask your doctor about adding strained or finely chopped meats. The palmar grasp usually develops between five and seven months, allowing your baby to handle finger foods like arrowroot biscuits or dried toast. By six months baby will probably have one or two teeth, but he won't have all his teeth for years. Don't worry. Babies can learn to chew even without a full set of chompers, but do serve food soft or chopped to make eating safe and easier.
	Yogurt, unsweetened	1–2 tablespoons	
	Vegetables, plain, strained	3–4 tablespoons	
	Meat, plain, strained	1–2 tablespoons	
	Crackers, toast, zwieback crackers	Small portion (½ ounce)	
	Iron-fortified cereal	4–6 tablespoons	
	Fruit juice, unsweetened, with vitamin C (but delay orange, pineapple, grapefruit, and tomato juice)	2–4 ounces	
	Breast milk/formula	24–32 ounces	

Age	Food	Amounts per Day	Comments
Nine to ten months	Iron-fortified cereal	4–6 tablespoons	Between nine and twelve months, move your baby away from strained fruits and vegetables and toward small servings of chopped or mashed foods. Increase the variety of table meats offered, and as the pincer grasp develops, increase the amount of finger foods served.
	Fruit juice, unsweetened	4 ounces	
	Fruit	6–8 tablespoons	
	Vegetables	6–8 tablespoons	
	Meat, fish, poultry, egg yolk, yogurt, cottage cheese	4–6 tablespoons	
	Crackers, toast, unsweetened cereal (including soft bread, bagels, rolls, or muffins)	1–2 small servings ($\frac{1}{2}$–1 ounce portion)	
Eleven to twelve months	Breast milk/formula	24–32 ounces	Encourage self-feeding, but expect messes. Offer a variety of foods, especially those rich in protein and calcium. Decrease breast milk and formula as you increase food intake.
	Iron-fortified cereal	4–6 tablespoons	
	Breads: crackers, toast, unsweetened cereal, zwieback	1–2 small servings ($\frac{1}{2}$–1 ounce portion)	
	Fruit juice; unsweetened with vitamin C	4 ounces	
	Fruit	$\frac{1}{2}$ cup	
	Vegetables	$\frac{1}{2}$ cup	
	Meat, fish, poultry, peanut butter*	$\frac{1}{2}$ cup chopped or 2–4 tablespoons	
	Potato, rice, noodles	1–3 small servings ($\frac{1}{2}$–1 ounce or 1–3 tablespoons equals a serving)	
	Breast milk/formula	24–30 ounces	

*Peanut butter: Some pediatricians wait until age two before adding because of allergy risk.

child to hold food with the fingers. You will want to allow your child to experiment with self-feeding at this time.

Simple Rules to Feed By

- Feed only breast milk or infant formula to drink in the first year—no cow's milk until after one year.
- Introduce some solid foods starting at four to six months.
- Add a good source of iron by six months (iron-fortified cereal, meat).
- Serve solid food pureed or mashed.
- Avoid hard round foods.
- Do not add salt or sugar to meals.
- Serve food warmed to body temperature.
- If juice is served, limit it to 4–6 ounces per day.
- Serve only one new food at a time, and wait at least 2 days before trying a new one.

REDUCING THE RISK OF A FOOD ALLERGY

An article in the *Journal of the American Dietetic Association* suggests introducing a new food every two to four days (two to three per week) as a reasonable rule if no history of family food allergies is present. If food allergies run in your family, try to breastfeed your baby as long as you can, ideally for a year or longer, and delay solid foods until at least six months; avoid dairy products until twelve months, delay eggs until age two, and avoid peanuts, tree nuts, and fish until age three. Always introduce only one food at a time, so you can identify any that are problematic.

If you are breastfeeding and your child develops a suspected food allergy, or your family has a history of food allergy, the AAP suggests you avoid cow's milk, eggs, fish, peanuts, and tree nuts in your own diet. (However, there is no evidence that eliminating these foods during pregnancy—with the possible exception of peanuts—is necessary.) Mothers eliminating some of these foods

may need a supplement of calcium and possibly vitamins. If eliminating these foods does not help, your health care provider may
recommend a hypoallergenic formula as an alternative to breastfeeding. A formula-fed infant with a confirmed cow's milk allergy
will need to switch to a hypoallergenic or soy formula, too.

Food Allergies

If you think food allergies are on the rise, you are probably
right. Approximately 6 to 8 percent of children under age four
have a food allergy, and 4 percent of all adults do as well.
According to the National Institutes of Health, peanut allergies in particular appear to be increasing, though no one can
say why. The foods most likely to cause a food allergy are
eggs, milk, wheat, soy, peanuts, tree nuts, fish, and shellfish.

PORTION SIZE

Portions are small in the first year. Not only are babies' stomachs
very small, but it is important to remember that in the first year
of life, most of their nutrients still come from their milk feeding.
The food they are learning to eat is a teaching tool and a source
of the important nutrient iron. A serving is only about one-quarter
the size of an adult serving.

WHAT TO EXPECT ABOUT GROWTH

Growth in the first year of your baby's life is phenomenal. After an
initial weight loss that occurs in the first few days after birth—
which is completely normal—your baby will regain her birth
weight by the seventh or tenth day, by four to six months she will
double her birth weight, and by one year she will triple her weight.
She will increase in length by 50 percent at the first birthday and
double in length by four years. Her stomach capacity increases,
too. While it is tiny at birth (able to hold less than 1 ounce), by the

first birthday it can hold about ¾ cup. Newborns' tiny stomachs make frequent feedings necessary.

Your health care provider will track your child's weight and length using standard growth charts. Growth charts are very useful to your baby's doctor, but they can be a source of both pride and concern to parents. Babies have different genetic potential and individual growth rates, so a child who is consistently in the 90th percentile for height and weight is not "healthier" than the infant who is consistently in the 10th percentile. Your health care provider will want to see consistent growth trends; any problematic changes will be identified at well-child visits, so keep those appointments. Weight gains in formula-fed babies are usually greater than in breastfed babies.

SPECIAL SITUATIONS

Feeding the Infant with Down Syndrome

Infants with Down syndrome can be breastfed, but poor sucking ability and other health problems may make breastfeeding difficult immediately after birth. If the infant is unable to nurse, expressed milk given another way should be considered. Ability to feed will usually improve within a few weeks, but it is critically important to seek the help of occupational therapists, lactation consultants, and other mothers with experience feeding a Down syndrome child.

For those families choosing formula, there is no special formula recommended unless there is a specific additional medical problem. If weight gain is slow, formula additives or special feeding tools may be advised. Reflux can be reduced by holding the baby in a semi-upright position and by keeping the bottle well positioned to prevent air swallowing. The baby with Down syndrome can be very sleepy, making the recommendation for feeding on demand much less applicable. To meet your child's nutritional needs, you will need to wake her every two to three hours, and nursing mothers may have to stimulate the breast with a breast pump to keep milk supply adequate.

With age the child with Down syndrome can follow the same

feeding schedule as other infants. However, hard solid foods that require chewing may need to be delayed, as tooth eruption can be slower, and teaching a child with Down syndrome to use eating utensils and a cup is likely to take a little longer. Your health care provider will use growth charts specifically designed for use with children with Down syndrome.

For more information, contact the National Down Syndrome Congress (www.ndsccenter.org), the National Down Syndrome Society (www.ndss.org), or La Leche League International (www .laleche.org).

Preterm Infant Nutrition

Aggressive nutrition from the time of birth is important in hopes that the need for catch-up growth will be less of an issue after discharge from the hospital. Also, what is fed in the early days and weeks affects long-term health. Most infants with a birth weight below 1,500 grams (about 3 pounds) will require parenteral nutrition in the first few weeks of life. When possible, infants can be fed breast milk, though this may need to be supplemented with a fortifier. Formula-fed infants will be given a specially designed formula rich in protein, minerals, nutrients, and essential fatty acids; such a formula usually continues until the post-conception date of forty weeks and often for an additional twelve weeks thereafter. Follow your hospital team's advice on feeding, as it will be most accurate and appropriate to meet your baby's needs.

Vegetarian Diets

Seven percent of Americans consider themselves vegetarian, but often parents wonder if their baby can be well nourished without meat. This is an important question, because the nutrient needs of babies are especially high and their rapid growth requires an excellent source of energy and protein as well as fat, vitamins, and minerals. Height and weight charts will be an important tool to assess your child's growth. If you are feeding your child a vegetarian or vegan diet and he is maintaining a growth rate appropriate for his age, you are probably doing just fine.

While breastfeeding or even while on formula, your baby will get plenty of nutrition, but as you wean your child food choices are critical. If your baby is not fed meat, poultry, or fish, you can substitute eggs, cheese, or yogurt and choose a cereal or bread fortified with zinc.

The following foods each contain 7 grams of protein, the amount in 1 ounce of cooked meat, fish, or poultry. Read more about proteins on page 31.

Egg, 1

Egg whites, 2

Parmesan cheese, 3 tablespoons (high in sodium)

Hard cheese, 1 ounce (high in sodium)

Beans, ⅓ to ½ cup

Soy flour, ¼ cup

Tempeh, 4 ounces

Tofu, 3 ounces

Nut butters, 1½ tablespoons (allergy risk)

Yogurt, 1 cup

Children who eat no animal or dairy products and rely on beans, cereal, nuts, seeds, fruit, and vegetables for their protein and energy needs will have a more complicated course. All of these are great foods, but for an infant it is the increased bulk of the vegetarian diet that makes it difficult for a baby to eat enough food to get all the calories and nutrients needed. Serve a good protein source such as beans, tofu, tempeh, or nut butters (when old enough) at every meal. Soy milk has a protein content similar to cow's milk, but rice milk is much lower in protein.

It is also particularly important to find a source of docosahexaenoic acid (DHA) and vitamin B_{12}. DHA is a fatty acid found in breast milk and now added to formula and some infant food. It has important health benefits, including brain and eye development. Outside of breast milk, DHA occurs in nature only in marine foods; it can be made in the body from alpha-linolenic acid, found in ground flaxseed, flaxseed oil, canola oil, and soybean oil, but experts are not sure how efficiently this is done. Algae-based supplements can be an acceptable vegan source of DHA. Eggs from hens fed marine foods can be a source of DHA for families eating a vegetarian diet that includes eggs.

Vitamin B_{12} is an essential nutrient found in animal-based foods, including eggs and dairy. Those who do not eat any animal-based foods will have to get B_{12} from fortified foods, such as infant formula, some brands of nutritional yeast, and fortified breakfast cereal, or from a supplement.

Here are some tips on how to provide a healthy meatless menu for your baby:

- Breastfeed or feed infant formula for the first year of life or longer.
- Serve your child enough food to maintain growth. Ask your health care provider for an assessment of your baby's growth.
- If you don't eat meat, substitute any of the protein sources listed above or on pages 31–32.
- Offer a wide variety of nutrient-dense foods.
- Include a good calcium source daily.
- Include a good source of the omega-3 fatty acid DHA.
- Get enough vitamin B_{12}.
- Include a good source of zinc-rich food daily.
- Include a good source of iron-rich food daily.

Recommended Supplements for Breastfed Vegan Infants

Vitamin K	Single dose given at birth
Vitamin D	200 IU (5 micrograms) beginning at three months for infants who do not get adequate sun exposure, live in northern climates, or are dark-skinned
Iron	1 milligram per kilogram (2.2 pounds) of body weight, daily beginning at four to six months
Vitamin B_{12}	0.4 microgram per day beginning at birth and

	0.5 microgram daily beginning at six months If the mother's diet is not adequate. Ask your health care provider for guidance.
Fluoride	Add after six months of age if water is not adequately fluoridated.
Zinc	Older infants may need additional zinc if adequate zinc is not consumed in food. Ask your health care provider for guidance.

Zinc and Meat

When I raised my children, meat was not commonly added to the diet until eight months. Now some nutritionists suggest we add it earlier because it is such a good source of zinc. Breast milk carries enough zinc for the first half year, but by seven months an alternative source is needed. Zinc can come from cereal, soybeans, lentils, peas, and nuts, but it is not easily absorbed from these foods because they also carry a substance called phytate, which inhibits the absorption of zinc. Traditional baby foods such as cereal, fruit, and vegetables are not great sources of zinc, either, unless they are fortified. On the other hand, 1 to 2 ounces of beef or turkey can supply an infant or child's daily requirement for zinc. Inadequate zinc may affect growth and appetite, and having enough of this mineral may be particularly important for low-birthweight infants. Babies need about 3 milligrams of zinc daily from seven months to three years. Formula is a reliable source of zinc.

Food	Zinc Content (in milligrams)
Enriched farina, ¾ cup cooked	0.12
Infant rice cereal, 1 tablespoon dry	0.05
Banana, 1 medium	0.18

Food	Zinc Content (in milligrams)
Peach, 1 medium	0.12
Carrot, 1 raw	0.35
Tofu, ½ cup	0.99
Beef, 3½ ounces	6.00
Turkey, dark meat, 3½ ounces	4.40
Egg, 1	0.55
Cod, 3 ounces	0.49
Baked beans, 1 cup	3.56
Wheat germ, ¼ cup	4.83

COW'S MILK AND LACTOSE INTOLERANCE

Cow's milk has no place in your baby's menu for his first year of life. Cow's milk is low in iron and hard to digest, causing tiny amounts of iron to be lost in the intestine and increasing the risk of iron deficiency. Stick to breast milk or infant formula in the first twelve months, and add them to infant cereal instead of cow's milk.

A milk-free diet is not the same as a lactose-free diet. Approximately 2–3 percent of infants will be allergic to the protein in cow's milk, and in these infants milk can cause constipation and gastroesophageal reflux. If milk allergy runs in your family, you will want to minimize milk and milk-containing food. Read labels very carefully for any terms that indicate milk or milk products, including butter, cheese, and casein. Note that goat's milk contains a protein similar to cow's milk, potentially causing a reaction in those with a cow's milk allergy. For more information on milk allergy, go to the Food Allergy and Anaphylaxis Network at www.foodallergy.com.

Some babies cannot tolerate the naturally occurring sugar called lactose that is found in milk and milk-containing products. A lactose sensitivity can be the cause of cramps, nausea, bloating, gas, and diarrhea, and it is treated by avoiding or limiting lactose. However, new research suggests that small amounts of lactose can be tolerated by most lactose-intolerant individuals, so try to establish your child's individual tolerance to lactose. Illnesses that cause diarrhea can sometimes lead to a temporary intolerance of lactose. Note that yogurt is often well tolerated by lactose-intolerant people, since the bacterial cultures used to make it produce some of the enzyme needed to properly digest the lactose. This is good because yogurt is a great calcium source.

Following a lactose-restricted or milk-free diet will require obtaining calcium from non-milk products. Read about calcium sources below.

Calcium and Lactose Content in Common Foods

Food	Calcium (milligrams)	Lactose (grams)
Calcium-fortified orange juice, 1 cup	320	0
Soy milk, 1 cup	200	0
Broccoli, raw, 1 cup	90	0
Pinto beans, cooked, ½ cup	40	0
Salmon, canned, 3 ounces with bones	205	0
Lettuce, ½ cup	10	0
Yogurt, 1 cup	415	5
Milk, 1 cup	295	11
Swiss cheese, 1 ounce	270	1
Ice cream, ½ cup	85	6
Cottage cheese, ½ cup	75	2–3

IMPORTANT FATTY ACIDS

Research over the past twenty years has explored the role of important fatty acids in infant health. Two in particular, arachidonic acid (ARA) and docosahexaenoic acid (DHA), are abundant in the brain and retina and are naturally present in breast milk (though the level fluctuates based on maternal diet). DHA is particularly important to premature babies to ensure good eye health. The AAP has no official position on supplementing infant formulas with ARA or DHA, but advisory groups from other countries recommend that infant formula, particularly formula for premature infants, should be supplemented with these fatty acids. Formulas sold in the United States that contain added ARA and DHA will clearly state it on the label. Read more on page 217.

VITAMIN SUPPLEMENTS

If you are exclusively breastfeeding your baby, starting at two months, your health care provider may recommend a vitamin D supplement. Our bodies make vitamin D when our skin is exposed to sunlight, and we used to believe breast-fed babies got enough vitamin D from sun. But with the use of sunscreens to reduce the risk of skin cancers, this may not be the case. In a 2007 *Journal of Nutrition* study, vitamin D deficiency was widespread among all new mothers. Even while taking a prenatal supplement containing vitamin D, women living in northern climates should ask the doctor about a vitamin D test. Formula is already supplemented with vitamin D, making an additional source unnecessary unless babies consume less than 16 ounces of formula daily. Older children and adolescents who do not get regular sun exposure and do not drink at least 2 cups of vitamin D fortified milk will need a supplement as well.

Another important nutrient that may need to be supplemented is iron. Approximately 9 percent of children under age three are deficient in iron, and one-third of these children have iron deficiency anemia. The risk of iron deficiency anemia can be reduced by adding a source of iron starting at six months. Most infants are born with enough stored iron to cover them for the first 4–6 months. If your health care provider suspects your child is at risk of iron deficiency, your baby will get a blood test to make sure iron levels are adequate, usually at nine to twelve months.

Never give any vitamin or mineral or other over-the-counter supplements used by adults to an infant unless specifically advised to do so. A baby's digestive tract is small and not well developed, putting a baby at greater risk of toxicity from supplements. Accidental poisoning caused by supplements that look like candy is not uncommon in young children—keep these out of a child's reach.

FLUORIDE

Two-thirds of communities in the United States have fluoridated water, and it has reduced the number of cavities in primary teeth by 60 percent. Fluoride reduces cavities by making teeth stronger and better able to resist the bacteria that cause tooth decay. Children living in areas without fluoridated water may be advised to take a supplement. However, it is important to accurately assess a child's intake of fluoride. Children may live in a community without fluoride in the water but receive child care in a community where the water is fluoridated. On the other hand, a child who lives in a community with fluoridated water but whose family drinks bottled water or uses certain types of filters might not be getting adequate amounts of fluoride to prevent cavities. With too little fluoride, teeth are not protected, but too much results in fluorosis, a cosmetic condition that can leave the teeth with white lines, a chalky appearance, or in severe cases pitting and brown staining. This is becoming more of an issue as products such as fluoridated toothpaste are used in combination with fluoride supplements or fluoridated water. For this reason many pediatricians do not recommend fluoridated toothpaste until after age two. Ask your health care provider for guidance—he or she will be well aware of this issue and know about the fluoride levels in your water supply. For more information on fluoride see www.cdc.gov/mmwr/pdf/rr/rr5014.pdf.

KEEPING YOUR BABY SAFE BY KEEPING A CLEAN KITCHEN

Your baby is more vulnerable to food poisoning and foodborne illness than an adult is because his immune system is not fully developed. Also, his tiny stomach contains less acid, and stomach acid can prevent harmful microorganisms from multiplying and getting into the digestive tract and causing illness. Soap and water is your baby's best protection. Use soap and warm water whenever you might be in contact with germs and to wash eating areas. Washing your hands after diaper changes and before meal preparation and feeding is particularly important.

Throw out any formula or food left at room temperature for more than one hour. Breast milk can be expressed and frozen immediately for up to one month or refrigerated for up to 48 hours. Keep those bottles clean! Always wash bottles with warm soapy water before refilling.

When you start solids, do not feed from the jar. Put a small amount of food in a bowl and refrigerate the rest until ready to use. Feeding a baby directly from the jar contaminates the food with your baby's saliva, which can carry germs that cause the food to spoil before you serve it again.

CREATE A POSITIVE FEEDING ENVIRONMENT

Right from the beginning, make mealtimes pleasant. Start with a smile. It lets your baby know that everything is okay even as she experiences something new. Remember, too, that messy is normal. Let your baby play with her food. A child needs to use her fingers—I promise she will learn to use the right utensils with time.

In the first four months, feed your baby on demand, but between four and six months start offering one meal of solid food per day. At six to seven months offer one or two meals. At eight months increase to two or three meals and continue that schedule until the first birthday. Be aware that it is normal for infants and young children to eat more at one meal and less at another. It is their way of self-regulating effectively. Again, parents' job is to offer food in a consistent, predictable manner, and it is the child's job to eat what she needs.

With a schedule, your baby knows she can depend on you to provide meals in a predictable manner, and she will not have to worry about food because you have taken care of it. You can help your baby be ready for meals by creating a routine she recognizes. Just as you have a rocker or chair you nurse in, have a feeding setup that your baby can identify with mealtime. Put her in the high chair, dress her with a bib, and give her a spoon to hold so she knows food is on the way.

A consistent sleep schedule will help mealtime go well. A well-rested child will be less fussy and able to concentrate on eating. Most babies need two (some three) naps every day. To make nap time go smoothly, establish a routine here as well. Take the child to her room, change the diaper, and then put the child down. Do this in the same order every day. Do not nurse or bottle-feed to get your child to sleep. Of course babies occasionally fall asleep while nursing, but if your child always falls asleep in your arms she will find it hard to soothe herself to sleep on her own. At night have a bedtime routine, too. A bath followed by a story or diaper change can all be part of a routine that will tell your baby sleep time is coming. Start between 7:30 and 8:30 and expect your baby to get eight to eleven hours of sleep (probably not consecutively).

FEEDING ANXIETY

There isn't one perfect way to feed your child. Some healthy babies started solid foods at three months; others were breast-fed exclusively until ten months. As long as you feed your child formula or breast milk, you can feel pretty confident he is getting a balanced diet.

In addition to the formula or breast milk, introduce a good food source of iron such as fortified infant cereal to the diet around six months of age. Then, as your child is interested, start offering new foods at a rate of one or two per week, avoiding the ones that could pose an allergy risk, as described on page 17. Keep your regularly scheduled well-child visits and his health and growth will be assessed by a professional who will alert you if there is something you should be doing differently.

Remember that your baby is an active partner in this feeding process. Give her too little and she will cry for more; give her too much and she might send it back at you.

The Value of Breastfeeding

If you are reading this book before your baby is born and are still deciding about breastfeeding or bottle feeding, I want to encourage the breastfeeding option. It really is the healthiest form of nutrition, and it's also both economical and convenient. Try to nurse as long as you can. Women who breastfeed their babies for at least the first few months of life may reduce their baby's risk of sudden infant death syndrome (SIDS), allergies, obesity, type 1 diabetes, Crohn's disease, and cancer. Breastfeeding appears to help infants be better self-regulators of food, meaning they can control what they eat based on how much they actually need. Proper self-regulation may be an important key to long-term weight control, a very important issue in an era where obesity statistics are alarming to us all.

The good news is that over 70 percent of mothers are breastfeeding for at least a little while but many new mothers still stop too soon. I have had several friends whose daughters have decided not to breastfeed at all or not for long. They tell me that their daughters feel vilified because they chose to use a bottle. No mother needs to feel guilty, but I have found that many of these women have not been supported in their decision to breastfeed. Well-meaning family members who share horror stories or ask undermining questions such as "Are you sure the baby is getting enough to eat?" are not being supportive. When I hear mothers tell me that breastfeeding "didn't work," I suspect many did not feel confident, and because they were worried about their baby's well-being they did what they thought was best and switched to formula. You should always trust your body and your baby. Breastfeeding works, but it can be hard in a culture that does not support it. If you have concerns, find mothers who have nursed their babies. As it has been for generations before us, the communal bond of mothers is essential.

Good Protein Sources

Protein is essential for growth, disease resistance, and healing injuries. Animal foods such as meat, poultry, and fish contain the eight essential amino acids needed to build and repair injuries. Plant foods, including nuts, beans, and grains, have a variety of essential amino acids that combine to make the same quality protein found in animal foods. The benefit of animal-based protein is that it carries a concentrated dose— about 7–10 grams of protein in 1 ounce, as compared to about 5 grams of protein in ½ cup beans. A child eating a variety of foods can meet protein requirements even if no meat is consumed.

Infants from seven to twelve months require 13.5 grams of protein daily. Children ages one to three years need 13 grams every day, and four-to-eight-year-olds need 19 grams.

Food	Protein (in grams)
Instant unsweetened oatmeal, 1 packet	4.4

Food	Protein (in grams)
Bread, 1 slice	2.0
Pasta, ¼ cup	1.7
Fruit, 1 cup	< 1
Peas, ½ cup	4.0
Tofu, ½ cup	10
Meat, fish, poultry, 1 ounce	7–10
Milk, ½ cup	4
Cheese, 1 ounce	6
Beans, ½ cup	5–7
Peanut butter, 2 tablespoons	7–8

How to Pick a Formula

All formulas are developed to replicate breast milk as closely as possible. The AAP recommends parents choose a formula with extra iron. Some of you may have heard that iron is constipating, but this is incorrect. Repeated studies have looked at the issue of iron and constipation and have found no increase in colic, constipation, gas, or fussiness associated with iron-fortified formula.

Some parents will choose soy formula as an alternative to cow's milk formula because their baby cannot tolerate cow's milk or because the parents want a vegetarian diet for their child. Soy formula is not recommended to prevent colic or allergy.

Do not boil formula; it can become too concentrated and hard to digest. Do not dilute formula to treat diarrhea; it won't provide enough nutrition.

Safe Equipment

Turn to the following resources to evaluate the products you buy for your baby and family.

Juvenile Products Manufacturers Association, www.ipma.org
Consumer Product Safety Commission, www.cpsc.gov

Childproofing Your Home

Start thinking about childproofing your home before your child can crawl. Go to www.kidshealth.org for a complete safety checklist. Do the obvious and important things, such as installing smoke detectors and window guards. If you are being given a baby shower, safety gates and safety netting (for decks and stairs) can be a great gift. And if you don't have a cordless phone, do get one—being cordless means you can follow your little one anywhere.

- Secure knives and scissors in a childproof drawer.
- Install a dishwasher lock and a stove lock.
- Add knob protectors to the stovetop.
- Keep chairs and steps away from the stovetop.
- Practice turning pot handles inward when you cook or use the back burners instead of the front burners.
- Childproof cupboards.
- Secure vitamins and all prescription and over-the-counter medications.
- Locate and secure any matches or lighters that are kept in the house.
- Keep cleaning solutions in a secure location.
- Secure cords from appliances and blinds so they are out of the baby's reach.
- Install outlet covers.

Poison Control

Keep this number in an obvious spot for you and your babysitters. I hope you will never need it, but if you do, you will want to have it immediately: 1-800-222-1222.

Be Prepared

When my children were young I kept emergency numbers taped to the inside of a cupboard door. The list included their doctor, police, fire department, my sister and mother, and my next-door neighbors. This can be especially valuable for babysitters.

Good Sources of Vitamin C

In the first year of life infants require 40–50 milligrams of vitamin C every day. Toddlers one to three years need 15 milligrams, children from four to thirteen 25–45 milligrams, and older children and adults 65–90 milligrams. Fruits and vegetables are the best sources, but it is the citrus fruits and juices and the fortified fruit juices that are the most reliable sources.

Food	Vitamin C (in milligrams)
Orange juice, 4 ounces	60
Grapefruit juice, 4 ounces	40
Apple juice, 4 ounces*	40
Grape juice, 4 ounces*	40
Strawberries, ½ cup	44
Melon, ½ cup	10–35
Orange, 1 medium	59

Raisins, ⅓ cup	2
Sweet pepper, ¼ cup	22
Tomato, 1 medium	23

*Apple and grape juice are not natural sources of vitamin C; infant juices have it added.

Good Sources of Iron

An infant seven to twelve months old requires 11 milligrams of iron daily; children from one to nine years need 7–10 milligrams. Boys over nine and men need 8–11 milligrams, and girls require 8 milligrams between the ages of nine and thirteen, 15 milligrams between the ages of fourteen and eighteen, and 18 milligrams from nineteen to thirty years. Breast milk and iron-fortified formula are the best sources in the first six months of life. When comparing the numbers below, keep in mind that the iron from animal sources is better absorbed than the iron added to cereal or found naturally in plant-based food, and serving a food rich in vitamin C with the iron-rich food enhances iron absorption.

Food	Iron (in milligrams)
Gerber infant rice cereal, ½ ounce	6.8
Instant unsweetened oatmeal, 1 packet	6.3
Bread, 1 slice	< 1
Fruit, 1 cup	< 1
Carrot, 1	0.4
Beef, 1 ounce	0.7
Chicken, 1 ounce	0.4
Egg, 1	0.6
Beans, ½ cup	0.7–2.4

THREE

Feeding Your Toddler

Your child is still growing significantly in her second year of life, but not at the same rate as in the first twelve months. For this reason, you are likely to see a natural reduction in food intake in the second year. This is normal—it simply reflects the decline in the amount of energy needed for growth. Your toddler will continue to develop her eating skills. By fifteen months she will learn to coordinate chewing, biting, and self-feeding and will become proficient at using the fingers, then a spoon, and even drinking from a cup. Encouraging your child to feed herself is a way for her to practice self-regulation, and this early age is the best time to learn it. When your child is ready, try serving liquids in a cup instead of a bottle. This way she learns to use a cup early, and it can prevent struggles later when you want to stop the bottle. During this stage, be prepared for messes, inefficient meals, and spills. This too is normal. When my children were in the fifteen-to-eighteen-month range, I kept a washable mat under the high chair to cover a rug.

After the first year children can move from an on-demand eating routine to a more structured routine of meals and snacks. It is not necessary that a child eat a lot at these times, just that food is offered and available. Feeding your child now in a predictable manner will make her feel secure, knowing she does not have to worry about when food will show up. By the time your child reaches two years she will be eating what the rest of the family eats. Your child will be well nourished if you offer her a variety of foods that match her developmental level. Now is also the time for you to model healthy eating habits. Practice "Do as I do," not "Do as I say." Just as in the first year of your child's life you needed to trust her to know how often she should nurse or how much she needed to drink from the bottle, that trust must continue now as she gets older.

Common Self-Feeding Skills

Age (months)

Milestone	4–6	7–8	9–11	12–14	15–18	19–24
Grasps food with hands	←———→					
Removes food from spoon with lips		←———→				
Feeds self using a spoon without spilling much			←—————————————→			
Drinks from a sippy cup		←———————→				
Eats food that requires chewing		←———————→				

Source: *JADA* (January 2004): S51

Child drinks from a regular cup without help

9–11 months	10%
12–14 months	14%
15–18 months	34%
19–24 months	57%

Teeth	
7–8 months	1–2 teeth
9–11 months	4–5 teeth
12–14 months	7–8 teeth
15–18 months	11 teeth
19–24 months	15–16 teeth

TEETHING FOODS

Around four months, teeth can start to emerge, and by age three all twenty primary teeth will be in place. To prevent cavities you will want to start keeping teeth clean as soon as they appear. A teething baby will love to put everything in her mouth. Ask your doctor about the use of products such as Orajel or Anbesol. These can give temporary relief but might also interfere with chewing ability because they cause numbness. This could be a significant problem because almost any food used as a teething ring, such as a bagel, can very quickly turn into a mushy, gooey substance that can be difficult to swallow.

Many parents turn to the Baby Safe Feeder. This is a baby-safe bag that holds the food and allows juices to be squeezed out but are too large to be a choking risk. These did not exist when I had my children, but they seem to make a lot of sense. I used a clean new sock filled with crushed ice and tied at the end instead as a teething ring. Cold chewy food can give relief, but when my girls were little I let them chomp on a clean damp washcloth or a clean adult-size toothbrush. Of course, never leave your little one alone while she has a teething food or object in her mouth.

The eruption of teeth is no reason to stop nursing. If your baby bites down while nursing, teach her not to do this by using your pinky finger to break her mouth's suction on your breast. Quite quickly a child learns to stop this habit.

To prevent the rash that often develops with the constant drooling that accompanies teething, pat your baby's chin dry as often as possible, and put a thin layer of baby oil on the chin to prevent irritation.

WHAT PARENTS WORRY ABOUT: FOOD

In your child's first year of life most of his nutrition came from the milk feeding; you introduced food so he could practice eating and to make sure he was getting an additional source of nutrients, particularly iron and zinc. Now in the second year it is important to lay the foundation of a good diet, and there will be many challenges. You may notice a decline in your child's appetite, and you are likely to worry about the limited variety in his diet. Parents worry that their child is too distracted at meals, dawdles, or craves sweets more than he should. It is important that you pay attention to what your child eats, but just as in the first year, your role as his teacher is essential. Your job is not to dictate how much to eat or force your child to eat a certain food but to help him learn how much he needs. You have to remember that your child is the only one who actually knows how much food he needs. Infants and toddlers are perfectly designed to self-regulate if you supply them with good food in a predictable manner.

According to the National Health and Nutrition Examination Survey, most American children do not meet the recommended dietary guidelines. The U.S. Department of Agriculture's Healthy Eating Index Score, a report card of sorts for the nation, finds that most of our children ages two to eight years "have a diet that needs improvement" or is "poor." A phone survey of more than three thousand parents found that up to one-third of infants and toddlers ate no vegetables or fruit on a given day. French fries were one of the top three vegetables for babies nine to eleven months old, and for fifteen-to-eighteen-month-olds french fries became the most popular vegetables. Though many infants were not eating the recommended amount of fruit per day, half were fed dessert or soda. These trends in poor food choices are very concerning because the food preferences your child establishes at age two to four probably predict his

What to Feed After Twelve Months

Calcium-rich foods: milk (plain whole milk, not chocolate milk), yogurt, cottage cheese, tofu, green leafy vegetables	2–4 servings	A serving is 4–8 ounces
Cereals, breads, rice, pasta, crackers	4 or more servings	About ⅓ of an adult portion
Fruit, no added sugar	2 or more servings	A serving is 6 ounces juice or 2–4 tablespoons fruit
Vegetables	2 or more servings	A serving is 1–3 tablespoons
Protein: meat, fish, poultry, eggs, beans, tofu, nut butter	2 servings	A serving is 2–4 tablespoons
Fat/oil: olive oil, canola oil, butter, margarine, mayonnaise	Use in food preparation as needed	

food preferences at age eight. According to the FITS survey (you read about this in Chapter 1), fruit drinks, candy, chips, and cookies were typical snack choices, along with milk, water, and crackers. Children given sugar-sweetened foods and drinks early in life consume more of these later as compared to kids not given these drinks early.

The child who does not learn to eat some fruits and vegetables will be eating a diet that puts him at risk of becoming overweight and increases the risk of heart disease, cancer, diabetes, and high blood pressure. You might be surprised to learn that despite these findings, most infants and toddlers are getting enough nutrition. This is true even for picky eaters and kids with slow motor skills. But getting enough of the nutrients we measure is not the same as getting enough of the foods that a child needs for optimal health. American children are not malnourished, but they are not well fed, either, and that is an important distinction.

Your child's nutritional future is in your hands, and now, after his first birthday, your family food choices matter. By fifteen months, he will know the difference between yogurt and ice cream, soda and water. You have to help him and protect him from eating a menu that is not in his best interest.

As I said earlier, toddlers should not be on a low-fat, low-cholesterol meal plan, but that is not the same as saying they should eat a high-fat menu. The fat that children get in food should occur naturally. For example, a toddler requires two to three servings of full-fat dairy products every day. Whole milk and whole-milk yogurt are natural sources of fat, and cooked chicken or beef also provide fat. But I would encourage a baked potato, a naturally low-fat food, over french fries so that the fat your child eats comes from food, not the cooking process.

Here is what a sample menu might look like for a one-year-old.

Breakfast	1 slice wheat toast
	1 cooked egg
	2 ounces orange juice
Snack	Apple slices
	2 ounces whole milk
Lunch	2 teaspoons peanut butter
	1 slice bread
	2 ounces whole milk
	4 baby carrots, sliced
Snack	¼ cup dry cereal
	6 grapes, sliced

Supper	½ cup cooked noodles
	¼ cup sauce
	1 ounce lean hamburger
	3 pieces cooked broccoli
	2 ounces whole milk
Snack	¼ cup canned fruit cocktail in water
	¼ cup yogurt

Other commonsense advice to prevent bad habits and accidents:

- Discourage bedtime bottles because they can lead to tooth decay.
- Insist your child sit during meals. This forces a focus on chewing and swallowing.
- Get rid of distractions while eating (or better yet don't start) such as TV or games
- Do not feed in the car. You may not be able to reach your child in time if he chokes, and eating is better encouraged as part of a family meal or focused snack.
- Avoid hard round foods such as hot dogs, hard pieces of fruit or vegetables, or round candy. Also avoid peanut butter in large portions (it can be sticky and hard to swallow).
- Offer cooked soft food.
- Avoid rub-on teething medication, which can cause chewing and swallowing problems when applied before meals.
- When you start using a cup, do not fill it to the top. Add only 1–2 tablespoons to start.
- Do not feed your child foods with artificial sweeteners. Your child needs real calories for energy.
- Avoid unpasteurized milk or juice, caffeine, and imitation foods such as nondairy creamers.

HOW GOOD PARENTS GO BAD

In the first five years of life children learn what and how to eat based on their culture and family feeding practices. The problem we have today is that our feeding practices, which have evolved over time, are based on a model of food scarcity. In the past, the threat of starvation was a real possibility. That threat does not exist today. In fact, the opposite is true. You are parenting in unprecedented conditions of dietary abundance, and you may not have adjusted accordingly. If you are a parent who worries more about getting your child to eat than what he is actually eating, your ideas about feeding are probably based on the outdated scarcity model.

See if any of the following sounds familiar. If your child likes a food, do you repeatedly serve it to the exclusion of other new foods? Do you cajole, coerce, and bribe your child to finish what's on his plate? Do you serve large portions or ask your child to clean the plate or finish his milk even when he demonstrates he is no longer hungry? If the answer is yes to any of these, your food models may be outdated.

This theory of feeding based on a scarcity model explains why some of the most loving and caring parents I know have been feeding their child a bad diet with the best of intentions. You can be at risk of becoming one of those parents, too. You are a normal parent if you worry about your child's unpredictable appetite, his preference for sweets, bad table behavior, or refused meals. If you find yourself fretting over your child's picky appetite even when your pediatrician reassures you his growth is on target, or if you won't try a new food because you fear he won't eat it, you may be headed for trouble. This is where you must trust your child to eat what he needs and feed your child a variety of foods. Keep in mind that the risk of giving your child too much food is a bigger threat for most children than too little.

As children grow they become independent eaters and develop a will of their own with regard to feeding. This independence is a very good thing, but our desire to see our children eat can result in feeding problems. Almost every parent I have ever talked to has a profound sense of relief and satisfaction when their child eats a meal robustly and with enthusiasm. Fifty years ago, when food choices were simple, parents fed what was on hand, such as a graham cracker, a slice of bread, or a piece of fruit. If a child did not like the choice, there was not likely to be an alternative, so a child ate what was given based on hunger. Children (and parents) were not seduced by salty, sweet, cleverly packaged treats. Today you can easily find something your child will like—freeze-dried snacks, yogurt-covered raisins, ready-to-eat macaroni and cheese—but should you? I think the answer is no. Offering your child what I call inferior foods, foods that have been stripped of fiber or processed with lots of salt or sugar, leads to overeating, and this is a problem even if the food is fortified with nutrients. In fact, the presence of nutrition claims on the label is sometimes a way to spot an inferior food. Instead, you want to encourage superior foods, foods that are minimally processed and carry a natural blend of fat, salt, sugar, and fiber. They will promote good growth and natural appetite control.

If you find yourself sliding toward a menu of limited variety, it is time to take stock. Get reassurance from your pediatrician that your child is growing well and start offering diversity. In Chapter 8 you will find a stage-by-stage guide filled with ideas and suggestions on how parents can feed their child effectively in this contemporary world of unprecedented dietary abundance.

PREVENTING OBESITY

Obesity is addressed here because it is on everybody's mind. Parents really do matter when it comes to obesity. You provide the genes and the parenting style, and you create the food environment. We live in a world of good-tasting, inexpensive food, and we eat anywhere and at any time. A child can become overweight in any family, and your child is at greater risk than any other generation in the history of mankind. Between 1963 and 1970 only 4–5 percent of children ages six to nineteen were overweight, but in 1999–2002 that figure increased to 16 percent. This increased risk is very real: 66 percent of adult Americans are considered overweight. Many mothers attribute their own weight gain to pregnancy, but research shows that all Americans, regardless of whether they have children or not, can expect to gain weight unless they eat well and move more. Your health care provider will be concerned, too, because excessive weight increases the risk of health problems that include diabetes, high blood pressure, cancer, and heart disease. Obesity can damage a child's self-esteem and have a negative social impact. If you are concerned about your child's weight, do not restrict. Instead, protect.

The rise in obesity has occurred because we are eating too much of the foods that do not promote satiety. "Satiety" is the word for feeling full; the feeling occurs when both hunger and appetite are satisfied. Hunger is the physical sensation that signals humans to eat and it occurs in response to a drop in blood sugar. Appetite is a psychological sensation, and it is linked to emotions, social cues, and the sight and aroma of food. Appetite may kick in even when we are full. For example, adults can eat a big meal, then see a delicious chocolate dessert and decide to make room for more. When we are sick we can experience hunger sensations but have no appetite because of the illness. Your child's satiety is influenced by a full tummy and the rise in blood sugar and hormone changes that signal fullness. Eating in response to true hunger is a good thing, but eating in response to appetite when not hungry is dangerous because it leads to overeating.

Your child lives in a world where food is available at almost every turn, and many of these foods are salty, fatty, or sweet. These do not satisfy hunger but are eaten in response to appetite. The foods that actually satisfy hunger and cause a sense of true fullness have plenty of water, fiber, and nutrients. Water in food is important because it adds volume without adding calories. Foods with a high water content include fruit, vegetables, low-fat dairy, cooked grains (such as oatmeal), and beans. Fiber adds weight but no calories, and foods that weigh more in our tummies tend to cause fullness. Protein as found in lean meats, dairy, and legumes also satisfies hunger. Unfortunately, many of the foods marketed to your child as snacks carry none of these important nutrients and therefore are not likely to satisfy true hunger, so be cautious.

The antidote to a food culture that is promoting foods in excess is the same simple principles that promote good nutrition. Eat three meals and planned snacks, and include a fruit or vegetable at every meal. At this early age obesity is not an issue, but poor eating habits are. Put the focus where it belongs. Do not restrict your child's menu, but do design it to protect him from overeating. You must eat well, too, to set a good example and for your own health.

It is important to note that many parents apply diet principles to their children that are more appropriate to a healthy diet for adults. Adult diet principles do not apply to infants and toddlers. In fact, they can be detrimental to their health. For most adults a low-fat, high-fiber diet will be an improvement because total calories are lower and nutrients are greater. The same menu for children can result in a calorie and nutrient intake that is too low, because the foods that are high in bulk will fill up a child's tummy long before they have met their nutritional needs.

The most important principle to focus on at this early age is variety in color, flavor, and textures. If a variety of foods are not introduced now, they are likely to be perceived as foreign and refused when older. If you follow these basic guidelines, you will be successful at feeding your child well.

- Start your child on a flexible but structured meal schedule—three meals and two or three snacks.
- Offer three or more different food items at every meal and make at least one of these items a fruit or vegetable. Include a fruit or vegetable at most snacks.

IDEAS FOR COPING WITH A PICKY EATER

By two years, as many as 50 percent of toddlers are described as being a "picky eater." I think that is because by this age they are aware of what foods look and taste like and they can express a preference for what is familiar and what they like the most.

Unfortunately, if kids are fed only the foods they are familiar with and like, they will be eating nothing but macaroni and cheese, pizza, and french fries. Toddlers are learning to eat and learning to be individuals. Being afraid of a new food may be a protective mechanism, and you want to respect that caution, but you also want to introduce your child to a variety of foods now because it will mean more variety later with age and better health. Please do not decide your child does not like a food until you have offered it at least eight to fifteen times.

In a study of the taste preferences of more than a hundred pairs of identical twins and a hundred pairs of non-identical twins, researchers found that the taste for protein-rich food such as meat and fish was inherited but the taste for fruit, sweets, and vegetables can be influenced by what they see others eat. This study suggests that children will learn to like vegetables only if they are served and the frequency of sweets in a child's diet can create a learned desire for these foods, the danger being that if kids learn to like sweets at the expense of more wholesome foods, their diet may be suboptimal. Quite simply, your child will learn to like a greater variety of food if you and the child's older siblings eat a variety of foods. Give your child the opportunity to be a good eater by providing the experience to try new food.

Praise your child for eating a new food, and do it when others are listening. One of the most detrimental practices is parents defining their child as a "picky eater." At this early age your child sees you as the ultimate authority, so if you define your child as a picky eater in front of friends and family, he is likely to prove you right. Instead, I recommend you reframe the description as more positive, for example, "Johnny is very particular about what he eats, but he is always willing to try at least one bite." Also praise your children's openness to new friends so they can overhear you.

Let him hear you speak positively about your own eating, too. I am not telling you to lie. Lots of parents I talk to confess they have their own food issues and don't like certain foods. Fish and Brussels sprouts are often cited as being unpopular. I tell them to be honest with their kids: "I'm trying new ways to cook because I know it's good for my health and other people tell me it's delicious."

Don't make a refused food mean something it does not. Too many times I have heard parents say their child is being difficult or willful because he has refused to eat a particular food. Young children love their mommy and daddy and want to please them, but they are also real people with their own likes and dislikes. If your child refuses a food, it can be because he is not hungry, he is not familiar with it, or he thinks it looks funny. These are just a few possibilities, but most likely he is not trying to be manipulative.

Influencing the Picky Eater

The British researcher Lucy Cooke has studied the effects of both genetics and environment on childhood eating habits. A study published in 2007 found that a large part of how our children perceive and accept food is inherited, but this trait can be influenced significantly by other factors such as seeing Mom and Dad eat a variety of foods and being repeatedly offered foods that were initially rejected. Dr. Cooke found that when parents were asked to expose young children to previously unpopular vegetables by offering small pieces every day for fourteen days, not only did the children increase how much they liked the food, but also eating habits in general got better and parents were offering other foods more often before giving up.

How to Cope with a Picky Eater

Coping with a child who does not like to try new foods is very similar to how you create a good eater.

- Stay on that flexible but structured schedule.
- Serve at least three foods at each meal and at least two for snacks, and make one of them a fruit or vegetable.
- Combine a familiar food with a new food.
- Trust that your child knows what she needs.
- Offer new foods eight to fifteen times.
- Don't force; smile and have fun!

Read Chapter 8 for more information.

FEEDING A TODDLER FOR GOOD HEALTH: PUTTING IT ALL TOGETHER

Now you know we live in a complicated food world. So how can we make it simple and keep our children healthy? Encourage your child's independence, but don't let her dictate what and when food is served. Only she knows how much she needs to eat at any meal or snack, but she really does not know what is good for her. In today's world innate preferences for sweet and salty foods can lead to very poor food choices, which are why you need to help with what is served.

Have a Schedule

The most important habit to get into is a regular meal schedule. Children are quick learners. If they know food will be served in a predictable manner, they don't have to overeat at one meal in case the next doesn't come on time.

Children do eat unpredictably, often more at one meal and less at another. If your child dawdles during a snack or meal (probably because he does not need to eat), he can make up for it at the next. Remember, toddlers need to eat fairly often, as their tummies are still quite small.

In the first year of life a loose schedule is established, and by the first birthday a regular breakfast-lunch-supper feeding routine with snacks should be established. Life can be busy, but don't worry—this schedule can be flexible. You don't have to eat at exactly the same time every day, though most kids do better if food is served on a reasonably structured schedule.

Serve Three or More Items at Meals, Two or More at Snacks

At meals serve three or more different food items, and at snacks offer at least two. Every food carries a different set of nutrients, so variety promotes nutrition. It also improves satiety and introduces children to new foods. A supper that includes only macaroni and cheese, for example, is not well rounded nutritionally, and it may promote overeating because it is so low in fiber and it offers no new taste experiences. Improve the quality of the meal by including a slice of fruit and some grated carrots. A snack that includes only a cracker does not introduce new foods and carries no protein or fiber for satiety. Serve a snack cracker with sliced grapes, mandarin orange pieces, or a spoonful of yogurt.

When I say to serve two or three items, I don't mean you should make your child eat all the items. I know food is not nutritious unless it is eaten, but forcing kids to eat makes them hate mealtime, and it is likely to make them want to avoid the food you are pushing. To help your child like new foods, let her see you eating the same foods she is eating.

Serve a Fruit or Vegetable at Every Meal and Snack

Offering a fruit or vegetable at every meal is a simple way to familiarize your child with the wide variety of foods that are available and increase the likelihood she will enjoy them. Eating fruits and vegetables bumps up intake of fiber and water-soluble vitamins and lays the foundation for a healthy food plan. Just remember portions are very small compared to adult portions. A child-size serving of fruit or vegetables is only ¼ cup.

Eat in a Designated Eating Location

Now is the time to start the habit of serving food in one designated spot, with no distractions from the TV or games. This is a very good habit for parents, too, as it prevents mindless eating in front of the TV or computer, one of the most significant causes of obesity in adults. It is much easier to prevent a bad habit than to break one. For most children meals will be in the high chair at the table; snacks might be served at a child-size table when the child is old enough. The child should be sitting while he eats; it will reduce the risk of choking and help the child focus on the business of eating. Always supervise your child while he is having a meal or snack.

Turn off the TV, sit at a table, eat the same foods as your child whenever possible, and create the environment you want now, before age two. There are so many demands on families' time that it takes a plan to make it happen. But family meals are critical to your child's well-being, now and in the future.

Be Thoughtful About What Your Child Drinks

If your child can drink milk, she needs approximately 2–3 cups per day. More than that can crowd out an appetite for other essential foods. Unsweetened juice is okay, but more than 6 ounces per day can lead to excessive weight gain, diarrhea, and poor nutrition. Instead of more juice, serve water and sliced fruit to satisfy thirst and provide nutrition.

Traveling Foods

When my children were little, I found it best to bring food with me while traveling. This way I always knew I would have good food they would like, and I supplemented it with what was on hand. When your baby is an infant you can freeze cubes of pureed food and put them in a cooler with ice packs, or use jarred infant food because of convenience and safety. For children who are a little older try ripe fruit and containers of yogurt in a cooler. A portable hand-operated food mill such as the one made by KidCo is an easy-to-use, easy-to-clean product that can turn table food into baby food almost effortlessly.

FOUR

Superior Foods

By now you know I think good food, a good meal, and fun in the kitchen is one of the best ways to spend quality time with your child. My goal for you and your family is to enjoy a variety of what I call superior foods—fresh, wholesome foods that still contain most of their nutrients. I hope that the information provided in this section will allow you to be confident in trying new foods and new recipes. I once had a client who, at age thirty-five, had never baked a potato and had absolutely no idea how to cook anything green. When she was a child in the 1970s her mother embraced convenience cooking: potatoes came out of a box, peas were always canned. She never knew what really good food tasted like, she did not know how to prepare it, and she had health issues as a result. Don't let that happen to your baby. Use this chapter to help you and your baby enjoy the pleasures of good food.

Let your child see you buying, preparing, and eating a wide variety of colorful and varied foods. When your child is older, let him help you make decisions about what to buy, and let him help cook. This is true quality time: it creates memories, educates, and improves well-being. Don't worry if your child is not a robust or adventurous eater. Just seeing you eat a variety of foods and being surrounded by good food will leave a lasting impression.

AVOID INFERIOR FOODS

In 1939 the Canadian pediatrician Clara Davis delivered a report on the eating behavior of a small group of children that she had studied for six years. Her study was intended to find out whether, if served wholesome foods, healthy children could select the right amount and types of food they needed without adult supervision. She allowed the children to self-select what they wanted and how much they wanted from a limited menu that included only fresh local foods—no canned foods, sugar, cream, butter, or cheese were included. Foods were prepared as simply as possible, and no salt or seasoning was added in the cooking. Bowls and plates were set on the table and nurses supervised the children for safety, but the children were given no guidance on what or how much to eat. Davis reported that "there were no failures of infants to manage their own diets, all had hearty appetites, all throve." She attributed the success of her experiment to the absence of "inferior foods."

Davis did not define inferior foods, but I use her term to describe foods that are the opposite of superior foods. In today's world, I would describe an inferior food as being heavily processed, having lost much of the original nutrition it started with, and often with significant amounts of added salt, fat, and sugar. One way to spot an inferior food today can be by the nutrition claims used to sell them. I know this might sound counterintuitive, but I have found this to be often the case.

Let me give you an example. The name of a popular infant snack food called Fruit Puffs implies it is a substitute for fruit. The label phrase "puffed grains with real fruit" would certainly suggest it is a wholesome grain food. Add the claim that it's a "good source of iron and zinc" and you can see why parents would want to try this item. It sounds like a terrific snack food. But a real piece of fruit will contain fiber, vitamins A and C, and potassium, and a true whole grain would add even more fiber. Unfortunately, Fruit Puffs contain no fiber, no vitamins A or C, and only 10 milligrams of potassium—an amount contained in 2 teaspoons of cantaloupe. Adding a little extra iron and zinc does not make up for eliminating real fruit and whole grains. Better to get the iron and zinc from foods that contain it naturally, such as meat and beans, or from a fortified infant cereal. Even more concerning to me is that the product virtually melts in the mouth, so the child does not learn to chew, and because this is a freeze-dried product, all the water has been removed. It is the water contained in superior foods that helps signal to your child that his tummy is full. I suspect that if this snack item or a food like it was part of Clara Davis's experiment it would have been so easy to eat and the sweet taste would have been so irresistible to the children that it might have caused her experiment to fail.

In preparing to write this book, I spent a lot of time in the baby food aisle at my local supermarket. Many new products have been added since I was there with two toddlers in tow. There are still many excellent baby foods, and organic items are numerous, but be wary of cereal bars, juice treats, fruit bars, and any snacks high in sodium or lacking the nutrients real fruit and whole grains carry.

HOW TO FIND SUPERIOR FOODS

All foods made by mother nature and minimally processed will be superior foods. Here are some guidelines for differentiating between superior and inferior foods. First, look for the products that use nutrition claims to sell the products, then use the labels to see if the product holds up to your scrutiny. See label on page 57.

Calcium

If a label claims a product is "made with real milk" or "real cheese," that implies it will be a good source of calcium. You can tell if it is by reading how much calcium a portion contains. A portion providing 100–160 calories should provide about 30 percent of the Daily Value for calcium, which indicates that it has around 300 milligrams calcium, the amount in 1 cup of milk. Prepared pudding often claims to be made with milk but usually contains very little calcium. And yogurt-covered fruit is really candy in disguise.

Fruit

A piece of real fruit (about ½ cup or a 70-calorie portion) will contain 1–2 grams fiber, vitamins A and C, potassium, and virtually no sodium. Compare a 70-calorie portion of food claiming it is "made with real fruit" to see if it contains the fiber and vitamins found in the real thing and if it has a significant amount of sodium. High sodium content alone will make it almost certain to be an inferior food.

Vegetable

Real vegetables have only 25 calories per ½ cup, almost no fat, 1–2 grams of fiber, and very little sodium (less than 50 milligrams). They also contain some vitamins A and C and potassium. Look at foods claiming to be "made with real vegetables" to see if they have fiber, and pay attention to the sodium content.

Whole Grain

An 80-calorie portion of any food said to be "whole-grain" should contain fiber, usually 2 grams, often more. That's equal to 1 slice of whole-grain bread or ½ cup brown rice or oatmeal. Of course the word "whole" as the first word on the ingredients list is another sure way to identify a superior food or look for the whole-grain stamp pictured on p. 56.

Protein

A 1-ounce serving of meat, poultry, or fish or 1 egg has about 7 grams of protein and some iron. A ¼ cup portion of beans or 1 tablespoon of peanut butter has about 4 grams of protein. A "good source of protein" should contain at least 7 grams of protein for a 50-to-80-calorie portion.

Sugar

The sugar listed on a food label includes both added and natural sugar, and it is often not a reliable indicator of quality. One cup of milk or plain yogurt contains about 12 grams of sugar, but this is natural sugar that occurs in all dairy products. A serving of dried fruit, such as ¼ cup of apricots, can contain 18 grams of sugar, but none of it is added. The sugar content can be useful when comparing similar products such as one brand of canned fruit or yogurt to another, and I find it very helpful when I buy cereals.

THE KEY IS BALANCE

I am not saying that you can't serve your baby or child fun or convenience foods. But many foods claiming to contain fruit and vegetables have lost the nutrients that are important to your child's health. The family that eats inferior foods at meals and snacks in place of fruits, vegetables, and whole grains will simply not be eating an optimal diet, and such a menu will increase the risk for poor nutrition and create a taste for highly processed foods. When you want to give your child some of these fun snacks, make the inferior food *one* of the items served at a meal or snack, not the entire snack, and pair it with more wholesome foods.

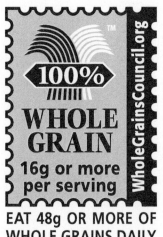

EAT 48g OR MORE OF WHOLE GRAINS DAILY

Whole Grain Stamps are a trademark of Oldways Preservation Trust and the Whole Grains Council. www.wholegrainscouncil.org

I am not against dessert, either, because sweet snacks and desserts are so abundant that you actually need to teach your child how to handle them. After your child reaches eighteen months, my advice is to serve dessert as part of a meal as often as you think appropriate (I suggest no more than once per day), and keep portions child-size, about 120–180 calories—two or three cookies, ½ cup pudding or ice cream, or a 2-inch square of cake. Read about discretionary calories on page 210.

Nutrition Facts

Serving Size 1 cup (228g)
Servings per Container 2

Amount Per Serving

Calories 280	Calories from Fat 120

	% Daily Value*
Total Fat 13g	20%
Saturated Fat 5g	25%
Trans Fat 2g	
Cholesterol 2mg	10%
Sodium 660mg	28%
Total Carbohydrate 31g	10%
Dietary Fiber 3g	0%
Sugars 5g	
Protein 5g	

Vitamin A 4%	•	Vitamin C 20%
Calcium 15%	•	Iron 4%

Percent Daily Values are based on a 2,000-calories diet. Your daily values may be higher or lower depending on your calorie needs

	Calories:	2,000	2,500
Total Fat	Less than	65g	80g
Sat Fat	Less than	20g	25g
Cholesterol	Less than	300g	300mg
Sodium	Less than	2,400mg	2,400mg
Total Carbohydrate		300g	375g
Fiber		25g	30g

Calories per gram:
Fat 9   •   Carbohydrate 4   •   Protein 4

Sodium Content Can Identify an Inferior Food

The tolerable upper limit for sodium has been set at 1,500 milligrams per day for children from one to three years (an upper limit for infants has not been determined). According to data released by the USDA in 2004, most young children under age six are consuming more than 2,000 milligrams per day. A high sodium intake is a concern because excess sodium can lead to high blood pressure, increasing the risk for heart attacks and kidney disease in later years. Sea salt may have a greater proportion of minerals than other types of salt, but it is still very high in sodium.

Eating foods rich in potassium can act as an antidote of sorts to sodium, but the same USDA report found young children consume less than 2,000 milligrams of potassium per day, though the recommended intake for one-to-three-year-olds is 3,000 milligrams and older children up to age eight need 3,800 milligrams. Foods rich in potassium include all fruits and vegetables.

To keep sodium in balance, read labels; prepared foods containing more than 400 milligrams of sodium per serving should be limited to once per day. Your child will get additional sodium naturally from milk and bread products and even from some vegetables.

COMMERCIAL BABY FOOD IS NOT AN INFERIOR FOOD

You might be surprised to hear that I do not criticize commercial baby food. I like it because it has no salt or sugar added, and even the non-organic baby foods are controlled for unwanted chemicals. It is also extremely convenient. I relied on jars of baby food when I had sitters taking care of my children and when we were traveling. What I don't like about commercial baby food is its blandness and limited variety, which is why I like parents to offer homemade food as often as they can. Start early teaching your child that there is a big world of food out there.

BE WARY OF ORGANIC JUNK FOOD

Just because it says "organic" or "natural" on the label does not mean it is good for your baby. Organic junk food is just as troubling as conventional junk food. In fact, it may be even more problematic because it lures you into a false sense of good nutrition—and it costs more.

SUPERIOR FOOD GUIDE

On the following pages my favorite family foods are listed alphabetically, with buying and preparation tips. The purpose of this
section is to inspire you to experiment with new foods not only for
your baby but also for Mom, Dad, and older children.

The phrase "buy organic" is listed next to the fruits and vegetables that should be purchased carrying the Certified Organic label.
If such products cannot be found, look for the country of origin
label and choose those grown in the United States. They abide by
the Environmental Protection Agency food safety laws. Read more
about organic food and country-of-origin labeling in Chapter 7.

The best way to prepare infant food is using moist cooking
methods such as steaming, stewing, or microwaving. Microwave
cooking is safe and nutritious if you use microwave-safe glass
dishes instead of plastic and always stir and test food before serving
to baby or children to even out any hot spots. Don't warm formula
in the microwave as bottles can feel cool to the touch but be hot inside. Use the Basic Baby Fruit Recipe, Basic Baby Vegetable Recipe,
and Basic Baby Meat Recipe in the next chapter for preparing small
portions for freezing.

At the end of each section, after the phrase "Family Table," you
will find suggestions for how to prepare this food for the entire
family. An asterisk (*) next to a recipe name indicates the recipe is
included in Chapter 6.

Apples (buy organic)

Apples are a good source of potassium and a particular type of soluble fiber called pectin. They have only small amounts of vitamin
C. The best cooking apples often taste tart when eaten raw but
cook into a lovely naturally sweet applesauce. Granny Smith and
Golden Delicious are considered good for both cooking and eating. Your baby will also love Cortland, Rome Beauty, Northern
Spy, and Winesap apples when cooked. Delicious, McIntosh, and

Pink Lady are great varieties to serve raw when your child is old enough to eat the skins.

Preparation. Simply peel, core, and chop. If there are bruises on an apple, just cut that part out. It will have no effect on the overall quality once cooked. To cook, add 1 tablespoon water or 100 percent fruit juice to ½ cup chopped apple and cook covered on the stovetop until tender, about 3 minutes. Make sure the liquid does not cook away. You can also microwave the apple, covered, for 1½–2 minutes (using the microwave yields more liquid). Drain and reserve the cooking liquid for use in pureeing. If you need even more liquid, use infant apple juice. Puree and strain for first-time eaters; for toddlers, just mash with a fork and serve. You will have about 4 tablespoons cooked applesauce. If the cooked apple tastes overly tart, mix with mashed banana or infant cereal to soften the flavor.

Tip. Most apples start to brown as soon as peeled or cut and exposed to the air. To prevent browning, cook right away or dip apple pieces into 1 cup cold water mixed with 1 teaspoon lemon juice.

Storage. Apples keep 2–4 weeks in the refrigerator. Use cooked apples within 2 days, or freeze puree in ice cube trays and keep for 1 month.

Caution. Apple skins could be a choking hazard for very young eaters. Avoid unpasteurized apple juice.

Family Table. All ages enjoy applesauce, Baked Apples,* and Apple Crisp.*

Apricots

These deep orange fruits are a very good source of vitamin A. They can usually be found fresh in late May and early June. They have a pleasant tart taste; the texture is similar to that of a peach, but less juicy. Apricots are picked ripe. Look for plump fruit with even color; they should yield when gently pressed, but avoid mushy apricots. Fresh apricots are fragile and do not travel well, but they are ideal for drying because the flavor holds up so well. Stewed dried apricots can blend beautifully with other fruits such as mashed banana and cooked pears. Many dried apricots are treated with additives to retain color and loss of flavor and vitamins. For infants it is better to read labels and avoid dried fruit treated with sulfur dioxide or sodium benzoate.

Preparation. For fresh apricots: Remove pit and chop. Apricots do not need to be peeled before cooking—the thin, fuzzy skin virtually disappears when pureed. In a small saucepan mix ½ cup chopped apricots (about two whole fruits) with 1 tablespoon water or 100 percent juice and simmer for 2–4 minutes, or microwave for 1 minute and let rest 1 minute. Puree in a food processor until smooth. For dried apricots: Chop ¼ cup dried apricots and add ¼ cup water. Simmer until very mushy, about 5 minutes. Or pour ¼ cup boiling water over dried apricots and let sit until mushy. Puree in a food processor until smooth, adding more water as needed. Cooked dried apricots are quite sweet and taste very good blended with yogurt or infant cereal or served as a dessert for you and baby when she is older.

Storage. Fresh apricots will keep refrigerated only 1–3 days. A cooked puree can last 2 days in the refrigerator, or freeze individual portions in ice cube trays or ½-cup portions for up to 2 months. Dried apricots can last in a cool dark spot for 1–2 months in an airtight container.

Family Table. Serve fresh, chopped in a fruit salad, or baked in Free-form Fruit Tart.*

Asparagus

Asparagus is hand-harvested, making it more expensive than many other vegetables. It is a good source of vitamins A and C, potassium, and the B vitamins. White asparagus is grown without exposure to the sun, and some consider it to have a superior taste, but it is less nutritious. The tips are particularly tender and best for baby; the stalk becomes tougher farther away from the tip. Look for thin stalks with tight, closed tips. However, even using the tenderest parts, asparagus does not easily blend into a smooth puree. You may want to offer asparagus when your child is older and on finger foods.

Preparation. Cut off the woody part of the stalk or use just the tips for baby and save the rest for you. Rinse and chop into ½-inch pieces. Place ½ cup chopped asparagus in a steamer and steam until tender, about 3 minutes. Or microwave for 1 minute and let rest for 2 minutes before pureeing or mashing.

Tip. Use only asparagus tips for pureeing.

Storage. Fresh asparagus can last 2–3 days before cooking. Once cooked, refrigerate for 2 days or freeze for up to 2 months.

Comments. If your baby likes asparagus, he may end up with smelly urine. Don't be surprised. Asparagus contains a harmless sulfur-based compound (related to skunk spray, of all things) that breaks down once eaten, and it makes urine smell funny.

Family Table. Steam and serve with freshly squeezed lemon juice.

Avocado

A very unique fruit that comes in a variety of shapes and sizes, the avocado ripens after picking and has heart-healthy fat. Most of the avocados we buy come from southern California. They are an excellent source of potassium and vitamins A and C. Babies and young children love avocados.

Preparation. Slice in half, remove peel and pit, and mash with a fork with a drop of apple juice with vitamin C or lemon juice (to stop the browning). No cooking is required; in fact, cooking can turn avocado bitter and alter the texture. Serve plain or mash with banana or applesauce.

Tip. To ripen, place in a paper bag with a banana. The banana speeds the ripening process.

Storage. Refrigerate only after fully ripened, with pit still in. Once sliced and in contact with the air, they start to brown; add lime juice, lemon juice, or another source of vitamin C to stop the browning, or wrap airtight in plastic wrap. Use refrigerated avocado within one day. Can be frozen for four weeks; remove the pit, brush cut surfaces with lemon or lime juice, and cover with plastic wrap.

Family Table. Serve cold in salad or as Guacamole.*

Bananas

Bananas are a very popular food for all ages. They are a natural source of potassium and fiber but provide only small amounts of vitamin C or iron. They are picked green and ripen in storage, and they spoil quickly once ripe. Plantains are a starchier type of banana and are served cooked as part of a meal, like potato or rice.

Preparation. Peel a ripe banana and puree with a little added water, formula, or breast milk. If your child is older, mash with a fork and serve as is. A 3-inch piece of banana blended with 1 tablespoon liquid will yield about 2 tablespoons of banana puree the consistency of yogurt. Bananas can also be cooked whole in the microwave; poke a few holes in the skin, cook for 1 minute, and let rest 1 minute more. The skin turns black but the inside is warm and creamy.

Storage. Keep in a cool dark spot, and refrigerate once ripe; the skin turns black in the refrigerator but the fruit inside does not discolor. Ripe bananas can be frozen whole in their skins and used in baked goods. See recipe for Banana Muffins.* To freeze pureed banana, mix with a little lemon water to prevent browning and freeze in ice cube trays for up to 1 month.

Caution. When serving as a finger food, slice lengthwise instead of into coins—this will reduce the risk of choking.

Family Table. Eat bananas raw or in baked goods such as Banana Muffins.*

Barley

Most barley sold in the supermarket is pearl barley, which has had the hull removed to speed cooking. It is inexpensive, widely available, and a good source of fiber, but not a true whole grain. Babies, toddlers, and children love this tender, creamy grain, and it deserves more space on our menus.

Preparation. Barley is slow-cooking, so this recipe makes a large portion. Freeze in single-serving portions for another time. Rinse ½ cup barley and mix with 3 cups water or Baby Broth (page 131) in a large pot. Bring to a boil, stir, reduce heat, cover, and cook 30–45 minutes, until tender. Do not expect barley to become as tender as white rice. It has a texture more like cooked oats. If you use whole barley, you will need to cook it longer. For babies, puree it; the grain will have absorbed a lot of water, and additional liquid will probably not be required for pureeing. It will have a texture similar to cooked oatmeal. It can also be served mashed or whole for older children.

Tip. Pearl barley is a fine addition to your child's diet, but it is not fortified with iron as infant oatmeal is. If your child needs extra iron, choose cereals and grains that have been enriched, meaning iron and B vitamins have been added to replace those lost in milling.

Storage. Keep uncooked barley in a cool, dark spot, like rice. Freeze cooked barley in single-serving portions.

Family Table. Serve barley instead of brown rice, or try Vegetable Barley Soup.*

Beans, Dried: Chickpeas, Kidney Beans, Black Beans, Navy Beans

Beans of all types are a great protein source. They are also a good source of the B vitamins and health-promoting antioxidants. Recipes containing beans consistently are listed as favorite infant and toddler foods. Serve plain or mix with cooked fruit or yogurt. When your child is older, try the bean recipes included in Chapter 5, "High Chair Cuisine."

Preparation. For canned beans: Choose canned beans with no added salt. Rinse beans and mash with a fork. For dried beans: Soak overnight in water. Drain, cover with water, and simmer until tender, 1–1½ hours. You can also try a pressure cooker for making beans; the Cuisinart electric model is very easy to use.

Storage. Once cooked, refrigerate and use in a day or two. Or mash and freeze for up to 1 month. Dried beans can easily last for a year or more in the cupboard.

Caution. Beans can cause gas because they contain a form of carbohydrate that doesn't get broken down by the body into an absorbable form of sugar. You can reduce this problem by soaking in several changes of water.

Family Table. Serve beans sprinkled in salads, sautéed with greens and garlic, and added to pasta. Try Imagination Soup,* Chickpea, Lentil, and Rice Soup,* or Turkey Sausage Soup with Beans and Greens.*

Beans, Green and Yellow

Yellow beans, also known as wax beans, supply less vitamin A than their dark green relative, but both provide vitamin C and fiber. Look for beans that sound crisp when snapped and have fresh-looking stems and tips; avoid wilted, flabby beans.

Preparation. Cut off stem and tip and cut into ½-inch pieces. Combine ½ cup prepared beans with 1 tablespoon water, cover, and cook on medium heat until tender. Or cover and microwave on high for 2 minutes. To puree smoothly, green and yellow beans must be cooked until very tender. Drain and puree with a little reserved cooking water.

Family Table. Steam and serve with freshly squeezed lemon juice.

Beef

Beef is America's favorite meat. Many pediatricians encourage the introduction of beef around eight months because it is a great source of zinc and iron; ask yours for advice. The highest grades of meat, prime and choice, are the tenderest because of their higher fat content; select beef is the leanest. Fat content varies by grade:

Prime: 10–13 percent fat | Ground beef:
Choice: 4–10 percent fat | 5–30 percent fat
Select: 2–4 percent fat

The protein and nutrient content for all grades, regardless of fat content, is very similar. In general, choose lean beef most of the time. All beef is an excellent source of protein, vitamin B_{12}, iron, and zinc.

Grass-fed beef is growing in popularity these days. It is leaner, with a stronger beef flavor.

Preparation. Puree ¼ cup chopped well-cooked beef until pasty, then add enough water or vegetable broth until puree is smooth.

Storage. Make sure all meat is purchased by the sell-by date. Refrigerate uncooked beef immediately in the package it comes in.

Whole pieces of meat can keep 1–2 days in the refrigerator, or freeze for longer storage. Ground beef should be cooked or frozen within 24 hours of purchase. Raw or cooked beef will keep in the freezer for 1–2 months.

Caution. Safe handling of beef is a serious issue. All beef must be cooked until there is no trace of pink to eliminate the risk of *E. coli,* a bacterium that can be found in any ground beef product (even naturally raised kinds) if not properly handled. Serve cooked meat in a form appropriate to age and chewing ability. Large pieces of meat can be a choking hazard. Read about hormones in beef on page 188.

Family Table. Grill, stir-fry, or roast the beef. Try Pot Roast* and Family Beef Stew.*

Beets

Beets are a good source of vitamin A, vitamin C, and potassium, and their rich red color indicates that they carry healthful antioxidants. Red is the most popular variety, but yellow beets are also delicious and the color does not bleed, making them much less messy to serve to little eaters. Beets have a reputation for being high in sugar, but this is only partially accurate. Beets are actually the source of 30 percent of the sugar produced worldwide, but that sugar is extracted from the juice of the beet. One cup of whole cooked beets has no more carbohydrate (the nutrient that breaks down to sugar) than is found in ½ cup of rice. Of more concern is that beets are a natural source of nitrates, which can be harmful to infants under three months. Read about nitrate poisoning on page 235. However, there is no problem giving beets to babies older than three months of age, since their digestive systems are more mature and can handle the substance. Beets are worth their long cooking time and the staining that may occur because they puree beautifully and children often really like their flavor.

Preparation. The greens on bunched beets accurately indicate freshness—avoid badly wilted or decayed tops on wilted, flabby beets. Cut off beet greens as soon as possible; this preserves freshness. The greens can be washed and prepared like spinach. Cover whole beets with water, bring to a boil, cover, reduce heat, and simmer 30–60 minutes, depending on size. Test for tenderness by inserting a fork. Beets can be cooked in 12–18 minutes in a pressure cooker. Once cooked, run them under cool water and remove skin with your fingers. Canned no-salt-added beets can be an easy alternative to preparing fresh beets. Chop cooked or canned beets and puree. Beets contain a lot of water, so additional liquid is not needed.

Storage. Fresh beets with tops removed can last a week refrigerated.

Caution. Beets can turn stool red because of the deep red pigment that gives them their color. This is harmless, but it can be alarming. Do not feed beets to babies under three months; read about nitrate poisoning on page 235.

Family Table. Serve boiled, as above, or roasted (page 171) and seasoned with salt and pepper.

Black Beans

See Beans, Dried.

Blackberries

See Raspberries.

Blueberries

These tiny fruits are packed with powerful antioxidants that promote good health. They are also a good source of vitamin C and fiber. Look for berries that have deep blue color and a silvery blush. This "frost" is their natural protective coating and it should not be rinsed away until just before serving. Large berries are grown commercially; the smaller, more tender berries are grown wild and usually available toward the end of summer or frozen all year-round. Avoid soft, mushy berries. Blueberries can be cooked and pureed, but the skins do not break down well and will need to be strained out. Once they are strained, you will have mostly liquid. You might want to serve cooked mashed berries to your child when she is old enough for more texture.

Preparation. Wash and pick over berries. Remove any stems or leaves. Rinse and serve raw when your child is old enough for finger foods. To cook, combine ½ cup berries with 1 tablespoon water or juice in a small saucepan. Cover and simmer for 2 minutes until berries burst, or microwave for 1 minute. Mash with a fork and mix with cereal or other cooked grain.

Storage. Do not rinse berries before refrigerating or freezing. Dry berries freeze beautifully and can be separated easily for use in cooked foods.

Caution. Baking soda, often used in baked goods, can turn blueberries green. This is harmless.

Family Table. Eat fresh or in salad. Try Free-form Fruit Tart* or Blueberry Muffins.*

Bread

Introduce whole-grain bread early so your child becomes familiar with it. Don't rely on color or healthy-sounding names alone when choosing bread. Instead, read labels. Whole-grain bread supplies approximately 2 grams of fiber per 80-calorie slice, and the word "whole" should be the first word in the ingredient list. Read about whole grains on page 110. Read about the whole-grain stamp on page 56.

More recently "white whole-wheat" bread has been introduced with the hope of pleasing consumers (and young children). Made from white wheat, it blends the milder flavor of white bread with the nutrient-rich qualities of whole-grain bread. White whole-wheat bread is as nutrient-dense as the traditional whole-wheat version.

Preparation. Bread can be served plain or toasted or used to make French toast or sandwiches when your child is older. Try my mother's recipe for homemade bread on page 150. It is almost foolproof and so delicious!

Storage. Bread without preservatives keeps best in the refrigerator. All bread freezes beautifully and thaws within minutes at room temperature or in the toaster.

Caution. Serve young children bread in small pieces. A large slice of bread can be a choking hazard.

Broccoli

Green broccoli is available year-round, and you'll occasionally find a purple variety and a cauliflower-broccoli hybrid called broccoflower. Broccoli rabe (not a true broccoli, but it looks so similar it shares the same name) has long, thin stems with broccoli-like flowers and a stronger flavor. Once cooked, they all turn green. Broccoli's deep green color indicates that it is a good source of vitamins A and C. Look for broccoli that has compact buds with deep color; tinges of yellow indicate overmaturity and loss of nutrients. Avoid broccoli that is not firm or that is marked with dark spots.

Because of its strong flavor, broccoli is not traditionally served as a baby food, but you can try it. Do offer it by eighteen months of age, as this is often a popular vegetable among older children. Many children like it cooked or raw as a cold finger food.

Preparation. Chop broccoli into ½-inch pieces. Flowers, stalks, and leaves are all edible (the leaves are very nutritious and flavorful). Combine ½ cup broccoli with ¼ cup water in a saucepan. Bring to a boil, then reduce heat and steam about 8 minutes, or until the stalks are very tender when pierced with a knife or easily mashed with a fork. Add more water to prevent burning if it looks dry. Puree with a little cooking water, or mash or chop finely.

Family Table. Steam and serve with lemon or a small amount of grated cheese.

Broth

Almost all canned broth is too high in sodium to be given to your baby. I recommend you make your own and freeze it in ice cube trays for the baby and in 1-cup or 1-quart containers for the family. If you can't make your own broth, look for low-sodium brands with less than 100 milligrams sodium per cup. I suggest no-salt-added broths from Health Valley or Imagine. See page 131 for broth recipes.

Brussels Sprouts

Brussels sprouts are little cabbages available fresh from October through December and frozen at any time. They are in the cabbage family and unfortunately are not universally popular, probably because of their strong, distinctive taste and their reputation for being "gassy," but let your child decide. For toddlers, chop or mash with a little butter or sprinkle with a small amount of grated cheese. They are an excellent source of fiber, potassium, and vitamins A and C. Look for Brussels sprouts with a bright color and tightly closed leaves.

Preparation. Remove loose leaves and trim bottoms. Cover whole sprouts with water, bring to a boil, reduce heat, and simmer 10 minutes or until tender.

Family Table. Serve with lemon or grated cheese. This may sound strange, but adding a little maple syrup to Brussels sprouts is the best way I know to serve them for the family. To prepare, parboil sprouts, drain, sauté in a little butter or oil, and drizzle with 1–2 tablespoons of pure maple syrup before serving. A grating of fresh nutmeg is a nice touch, too.

Buckwheat

Buckwheat is available as roasted groats (often called kasha), as flour for use in pancakes and other baked goods, and as noodles (soba). Despite its name, buckwheat does not contain wheat. It is gluten-free.

Preparation. This method can be used to prepare kasha for children one year and older who are eating eggs. Heat 1 cup of Baby Broth (page 131) to a boil. Set aside. In a bowl, mix together ½ cup kasha and 1 egg until completely blended. In a small saucepan melt 1 tablespoon butter. Add kasha-egg mixture and cook for 2–3 minutes, until the kernels look dry and have separated. Pour in the hot liquid and simmer, covered, until tender, about 5 minutes. Serve instead of brown rice.

Bulgur

Bulgur is cracked wheat that has been parboiled and dried for storage. You may know it best as the primary ingredient in tabbouleh, a popular Middle Eastern cold salad of bulgur, herbs, olive oil, and lemon. It has a nutty flavor and is at its best combined with other ingredients in soups or used to replace ground meat in chili.

Family Table. Try Quick-Cooking Chili.*

Cabbage

There are several types of cabbage, including green cabbage, red cabbage, and Savoy cabbage. There are also several types of Chinese cabbage (often called Napa cabbage). All can be substituted in any cabbage recipe. Red takes longer to cook, but all make yummy salads for the family table. Cabbage supplies vitamins A and C, fiber, and potassium as well as small amounts of many other nutrients. Look for cabbage that is firm with healthy-looking leaves. It is okay if the outermost leaves are loose, as these are usually discarded before cooking. Cabbage is not a traditional baby food. It has a reputation for being gassy and it takes a while to cook. Because there are so many other colorful vegetables to choose from, many parents avoid it.

Storage. A head of cabbage can last 1–2 weeks in the refrigerator. Cooked cabbage does not freeze well.

Family Table. Coleslaw or Stuffed Cabbage.*

Canola Oil

See Cooking Oils and Other Dietary Fats.

Cantaloupe

See Melon.

Carrots (buy organic)

Available year-round and a very popular vegetable among children. Carrots are a fabulous source of vitamin A and fiber. Look for carrots that are firm with smooth, well-colored skin. The tops, if still attached, should be fresh and a deep green color. Trim greens before refrigerating to prolong storage. Avoid carrots that do not feel crisp or that have a green tinge.

Preparation. Scrub under running water. Peel if the outer skin is a little bitter. Chop into ¼-inch chunks. Place ⅔ cup prepared carrots in a saucepan with 2 tablespoons water or vegetable broth. Bring to a boil, reduce heat, and cook until tender, about 2–4 minutes. Or microwave, covered, for 1½ minutes and let rest for 2 minutes. The carrots are done if they can be easily mashed with a fork or pierced with a knife. If they are not thoroughly cooked, they will not puree smoothly. Puree with the cooking water until smooth or mash with a fork for older eaters.

Storage. Fresh carrots can last 1–2 weeks in the refrigerator. Once cooked, use within 2 days, or freeze purees for up to 1 month.

Caution. When your child is ready for raw finger foods, serve carrots grated, not as coins, and do not use a whole carrot as a teething food. A chunk of hard carrot can easily become a choking hazard. All carrots can be a source of nitrates; read about nitrate poisoning on page 235.

Family Table. Boil, steam, microwave, or pressure-cook. Use in stews, in casseroles, and grated in salads.

Cauliflower

This creamy white vegetable has a strong flavor and is a good source of vitamin C. Many parents think their child will not like it, but don't make that assumption until you've offered it several times. It tastes best when mashed with a little bit of butter or mixed with cooked carrots. It is available fresh almost year-round. Look for cauliflower heads that are compact and creamy white, with no black spots. If the outer leaves are attached, they should be a fresh green color. Green or purple varieties taste and cook like white cauliflower.

Preparation. Divide the cauliflower florets into small pieces or chop with a knife. Discard the center core, as it is usually tough. Place ½ cup chopped cauliflower in a small saucepan. Add water to cover, bring to a boil, and simmer 3–4 minutes, until tender. Or microwave, covered, for 2 minutes and rest for 1 minute. Puree with a little cooking water, mash, or cool and serve as a finger food.

Tip. Pureeing or mashing cauliflower enhances flavor and has the secondary benefit of reducing its potential for causing gas, a problem some (but not all) adults report.

Storage. Fresh cauliflower will last up to a week in the refrigerator. When the florets start to spread, it indicates aging.

Family Table. Steam, boil, or roast. To serve, sprinkle with parmesan cheese or a drizzle of garlic-infused olive oil (made by simmering garlic in oil). Many adults use mashed cauliflower as a delicious low-calorie substitute for mashed potato; you can also combine mashed potato with mashed cauliflower.

Celery (buy organic)

Celery is a good source of fiber and when sautéed or chopped adds a lot of flavor to dishes at the family table. It is not a baby food because the strings could be a choking hazard, and it is not a nutrition powerhouse. It can be a terrific snack food for older children. For example celery with peanut butter is always a favorite after school. Look for bunches of celery that have a solid feel and clean glossy color.

Preparation. Rinse, peel with a vegetable peeler, chop, and serve raw to older children.

Storage. Celery can last quite a long time in the refrigerator. If it becomes wilted, it can be refreshed by standing freshly cut stalks in water.

Family Table. Celery is a great flavor enhancer chopped in salads or cooked into stews. It's a terrific no-calorie snack.

Cheese

Children love cheese, and many parents offer cottage cheese or sliced cheese starting at around eight months. Cheese is a good food, but you don't want it to crowd out other good foods. It becomes a favorite because of its naturally high salt and fat content. Choose lower-salt cheeses such as hard cheese instead of American cheese, and then mix up the protein choices you serve your child. At meals alternate cheese with cooked meat, poultry, yogurt, tofu, or beans. When you do serve cheese, don't serve it with other high-salt foods such as saltines. Instead, pair it with fresh fruit or cooked vegetables. Cheese does not need to be cooked. If wrapped and stored properly, it can last for 4 weeks in the refrigerator. When buying ricotta and cottage cheese, look at the sell-by date.

Compare the protein, calcium, and sodium in cheese and cheese alternatives to other dairy and calcium sources:

Cheddar or mozzarella (1 ounce): 7 grams protein, 200 milligrams calcium, 170 milligrams sodium

American cheese (1 ounce): 6 grams protein, 174 milligrams calcium, 406 milligrams sodium

Milk (1 cup): 8 grams protein, 300 milligrams calcium, 129 milligrams sodium

Chicken (1 ounce): 7 grams protein, 3 milligrams calcium, 30 milligrams sodium

Cottage cheese (1 cup): 6 grams protein, 150 milligrams calcium, 900 milligrams sodium

Yogurt (1 cup): 8 grams protein, 300 milligrams calcium, 100 milligrams sodium

Tofu (½ cup firm): 20 grams protein, 300 milligrams calcium, 18 milligrams sodium

Cherries (buy organic)

Sweet cherries find their way to market from May to August and are a great source of potassium. They are not a traditional infant food, because other foods that are easier to find and prepare like peaches and bananas crowd them out, but older children love them when they can remove the pit by themselves. They are picked ripe. Look for very dark, plump fruit with glossy skin and attached stems. Sour cherries are usually sold canned in pie filling.

Preparation. Wash, pit, and serve chopped.

Storage. Keep refrigerated. Can be frozen.

Caution. Be sure to remove pits before serving.

Family Table. Serve in fruit salads, or try Cherry Clafouti.*

Chicken

Chicken is a great protein source. The dark meat contains the most iron. It's a perennially popular food, and a good choice for babies ready for meat.

Preparation. See Baby's First Chicken, page 119. To poach a single piece of chicken for pureeing, cover one boneless, skinless chicken breast with water. Add a whole bay leaf and simmer for 20 minutes or until cooked through. Remove the bay leaf. Chop the meat and puree, or finely chop depending on age.

Caution. The potential for salmonella poisoning has become such a serious concern that poultry carries safe handling guidelines on the label. Even organic and free-range chicken must be handled properly. Heed the safety warnings and cook poultry thoroughly, until the dark meat reaches 180°F and the white meat 170°F.

Storage. Use uncooked chicken within 24 hours or freeze it. Cooked chicken should be used within 2 days. Once you puree chicken, freeze any leftover in ice cube trays for another meal.

Family Table. Roast Chicken.*

Chickpeas

See Beans, Dried.

Clementine

These small fruits with loose skins also go by the name mandarin oranges. They are easy to peel and are usually eaten raw. Canned, no-sugar-added versions are also a convenient alternative. Look for fruit that feels firm and has a bright yellow-orange color. They can be kept at room temperature for two to three days, then must be refrigerated. See "Oranges" for more information.

Preparation. Peel, separate into small sections, and chop for toddlers. Not a recommended infant food because they are so fibrous.

Family Table. They are a perfect size for a snack. Or use raw in fruit salad.

Cod

See Fish.

Cooking Oils and Other Dietary Fats

Choosing the right cooking oil and deciding between butter and margarine can be confusing because there have been so many health issues and conflicting claims made about many of them. To make your own decision, consider the following information.

All cooking oils and dietary fats are made up of a combination of saturated, monounsaturated, and polyunsaturated fatty acids. Polyunsaturated fatty acids include both omega-6 fatty acids and omega-3 fatty acids. These two fatty acids can protect the heart. However, many nutritionists believe we get too many omega-6-containing fats (found in grapeseed oil, soybean oil, peanut oil, and the store-bought foods made with them) and not enough omega-3 fatty acids (found in canola oil, flaxseed oil, and oil from cold-water fish). Good sources of monounsaturated fats include olive oil, hazelnut oil, almond oil, and canola oil. Canola oil is a good source of both mono- and polyunsaturated fats. Oils with a high percentage of polyunsaturated fat include safflower oil, sunflower oil, and corn oil. Fats that have a high saturated fat content are solid at room temperature and can raise blood levels of LDL cholesterol, increasing the risk of heart disease. Such fats include coconut oil, palm kernel oil, cocoa butter, butter, palm oil, beef tallow, lard, and chicken fat. Avoid these or use them judiciously for flavor. Fats and oils with a high polyunsaturated fat content can lower cholesterol.

Some of you may have heard concerns about canola oil containing erucic acid, which cannot be easily broken down by the digestive systems of unweaned babies. Canola oil is made from rapeseed, and prior to 1974, rapeseed oil carried high levels of erucic acid. The oil we know as canola oil today (the name is actually a trademark) is made from rapeseed that has a very low level of erucic acid and is safe to consume.

Trans fats are created by manufacturers from liquid oils to make solid fats that are more stable and less likely to become rancid. Some trans fat occurs naturally in meat, dairy products, and tropical oils. They behave like saturated fat and increase heart disease risk so you will want to avoid them. As of January 2006, trans fat content has been listed on labels and as a result removed from most products when possible.

My suggestion is to choose oils and fats harvested from plants. I suggest canola oil for cooking, olive oil for flavor, and soft margarine containing no trans fats and low in saturated fat for an everyday spread, or use real butter in small amounts. When shopping for cooking oils, be aware that the term "expeller pressed" means the oil comes from the first pressing and is extracted at a low temperature, which preserves the most flavor.

Do not use margarine fortified with plant stanols/sterols on a regular basis for babies and young children. These natural plant chemicals are added to some margarines to lower cholesterol in adolescents and adults, and can be very beneficial. However, there is some concern that these chemicals could block the absorption of fat-soluble vitamins in very young children. I don't recommend Enova oil for babies, either. This oil was developed in 1999 and is not absorbed efficiently in the small intestine. Some adults use it in the hope it will control weight and lower fat levels in the blood.

Corn

Corn is not served as infant food because it can be hard to digest. Many families wait until a child is eight months or older before offering it, and then it often becomes a favorite. America's largest food crop (though most of it is fed to livestock), corn is a great source of fiber, and yellow corn is a good source of vitamin A.

Look for corn that has been kept cold after picking. The ear should feel plump and heavy, with the husks green in color and the silk moist-looking. Avoid ears with underdeveloped kernels.

Preparation. Cut kernels from the cob by running a sharp knife down the side. The kernels come off in sheets. Place the raw kernels in a saucepan and cover with a small amount of water or vegetable broth. Simmer for 2 minutes, until tender. To microwave corn, place the entire ear including the husk in the microwave and cook for 1–2 minutes until the ear is hot to the touch. Allow it to cool before removing the silk and husk. Serve corn when your child is older and eating finger foods or able to chew right from the cob.

Storage. Use fresh corn within a day.

Caution. Popcorn is not be served to infants or young toddlers because of the choking risk.

Family Table. Serve corn fresh on the cob or prepared as above without pureeing. Frozen corn is a satisfactory and convenient alternative to fresh corn kernels.

Cornmeal (Polenta)

This is a treat and many children love it. Serve whole cornmeal or enriched cornmeal as a hot porridge, or use it to replace some of the flour when making muffins or pancakes. It can be a good source of fiber and B vitamins. It comes in white or yellow varieties. Whole cornmeal has a fuller taste but can go stale faster.

Preparation. Bring 1 cup water to a boil and stir in ¼ cup whole cornmeal. Reduce heat and cook, stirring constantly, until thick. Serve with milk or pureed fruit.

Tip. Older cornmeal may take longer to cook because it has lost more moisture.

Storage. Whole-grain cornmeal should be refrigerated or frozen to prolong freshness.

Family Table. Make polenta with 1 cup cornmeal and 4 cups water, and add a pinch of salt. Cook, stirring until smooth. Top with tomato sauce. Or try Polenta with Cheese and Roasted Vegetables.* Use cornmeal in Corn Muffins* or to make Cornmeal Pancakes.*

Couscous

Most couscous sold in the supermarket is instant and not a whole grain, unless the words "whole grain" are clearly listed. It is made from semolina wheat flour that is shaped into granules, so it is actually a pasta. The preferred starch in North Africa, it is a delicious, quick-cooking side dish that your child is likely to enjoy. Jerusalem couscous is a larger size that takes a little longer to cook.

Preparation. Pour ½ cup couscous into a small saucepan and add enough boiling water to cover, about 1 cup. Bring to a boil, stir once, cover, turn off heat, and let stand 5 minutes. Fluff before serving. Serve in place of polenta, rice, or potato. Mash or serve as a finger food at nine to ten months. Mix with milk, yogurt, or cottage cheese when your child is older and eating these dairy foods.

Family Table. Prepare as above and top with cooked meat, roasted vegetables, or Italian meat sauce, or use in place of pasta to make a cold salad.

Cranberries

Cranberries keep well and are abundant in the winter months. They are naturally sour and are usually prepared with a large amount of sugar and served as a cranberry sauce. Some cooks have successfully sweetened them with fruit juice, but in general I would not recommend them for babies. Dried cranberries have gained popularity as an addition to cold salads, but they, too, have large amounts of sugar added. Cranberry juice is not a recommended infant juice because of its high sugar content.

Cucumbers

These are most abundant in the summer months and taste best when eaten fresh from the vine. Look for cucumbers that are firm with a good green color, and choose ones that are not too large. A withered skin indicates that they are old. If the skin has not been waxed, adults can wash cucumbers and eat them with the skin on. They are not a rich source of nutrition, and they are extremely low in calories because they are 96 percent water. Not recommended for infants, but a good snack food for older toddlers.

Preparation. Peel and slice into quarters, scrape out the seeds, and chop into finger food or blend with cold yogurt and serve with a spoon.

Storage. Depending on age, a cucumber can last 4–5 days in the refrigerator.

Family Table. Use in salads or mix with yogurt, dill, and lemon for a healthful summer salad.

Edamame

See Soybeans.

Eggplant

Thomas Jefferson introduced this vegetable to America. Eggplant contains fiber and potassium and very few calories. Look for eggplants that feel firm and heavy. They should not be brown or shriveled, and when pressed the skin should bounce back with no indentation remaining.

Tip. Large eggplants can sometimes be bitter, but if you buy small eggplants, they can be cooked with the skin on, and they won't need to be salted to draw out the bitterness.

Storage. Eggplant can keep for 3–4 days refrigerated.

Family Table. Serve as eggplant parmesan, try it roasted (page 171), or prepare Eggplant Caviar.*

Eggs

Eggs are packed with nutrition, but parents may be concerned about three issues: cholesterol, salmonella, and humane treatment of hens. These issues can be managed effectively with a little bit of knowledge.

All eggs carry cholesterol, but it is saturated fat that is a concern. One egg has less than 2 grams saturated fat. Serve your baby eggs but hold the bacon, sausage, and cheese, which do far more harm.

Salmonella is a dangerous bacterium, so cook eggs thoroughly, and don't let raw egg touch foods that will not be cooked before eating, countertops used for food preparation, or utensils. Always wash your hands after handling raw eggs. Look for eggs with the Certified Humane seal (see page 188) and you will know the hens that laid them have had a decent life.

Preparation. Hard-boil in the shell, poach, or scramble. Puree cooked egg yolk with breast milk or formula, or mash with a fork. Try combining it with cooked vegetable or fruit.

Tip. Most parents wait until nine months to add egg yolk and twelve months to add egg white to baby's menu. Egg white is almost pure protein and the part most likely to cause an allergy if your baby is susceptible to an egg allergy. Egg substitute, sold in cartons or frozen, is made almost entirely of egg white and so is not recommended for babies under twelve months. I do, however, use these pasteurized egg substitutes when baking with older children, because the pasteurization eliminates the risk of salmonella poisoning and I don't have to worry when they lick the bowl. Eggs from hens fed a diet including fish oil, algae, or flaxseed have more of the omega-3 fatty acid called DHA, about 50–150 milligrams in each egg.

Storage. Keep eggs refrigerated in the carton they were purchased in.

Figs

Figs are available fresh in the spring and dried year-round. Fresh figs have a thin skin that is easy to peel. Look for fruit with smooth, plump skin. It should feel firm in the hand, not mushy. Fresh figs are a good source of fiber and potassium and small amounts of minerals.

Preparation. Fresh figs can be eaten raw. Babies probably will not like the texture of the tiny seeds, so serve figs as finger foods when children are older, or mash a ripe fig and mix with cereal. Dried figs can be eaten like raisins. Chop into small pieces that won't cause choking.

Storage. Once ripe, fresh figs should be refrigerated and used within a day or so. Dried figs can last a month or more if kept in a cool dark spot. Look for dried figs that contain no sulfites or sodium benzoate.

Family Table. Serve fresh figs as a delicious snack. Or cut in half, lightly brush with oil, skewer, and grill; serve alongside your favorite meats and vegetables or at the end of a barbecue with a dollop of good ice cream.

Fish

Fish is a superior food and should be part of your child's diet. Children often like lean white fish fillets such as haddock or cod. Oily fish, including bluefish, salmon, trout, swordfish, and tuna, have a stronger taste but more health benefits. They contain the polyunsaturated omega-3 fatty acids called eicosapentaenoic acid (EPA) and docosahexaenoic acid (DHA), which reduce the cholesterol the liver makes and help prevent plaque buildup. Children who eat fish also have a lower incidence of asthma.

Currently there are serious concerns about contamination of certain types of fish by PCBs, dioxin, and mercury, raising the question of whether the health benefits of the omega-3 fatty acids outweigh the risk from contaminants. The Environmental Protection Agency has advised that young children not be given shark, swordfish, king mackerel, and tilefish because they can contain high levels of mercury. Shrimp, canned light tuna, salmon (wild), pollock, and catfish are all low in mercury. Choose canned light tuna over albacore (white) tuna. For more information on mercury in fish, go to www.cfsan.fda.gov/~frf/sea-mehg.html.

If you want to serve your child canned tuna for the health benefits but worry about health risks, limit the amount you serve to 2 ounces of canned light tuna per week. This is a small amount of fish, but it can contain more than 350 milligrams of DHA, a significant amount.

Besides contaminants, there are concerns about how fish farming harvesting and practices impact the environment. Environmental Defense has compiled a list of the best fish based on nutrition and environmental contaminants. This is one of the best resources to make sense of this confusing issue. A list of their recommended fish is provided below, and a very handy pocket guide can be printed from their Web page. I recommend you keep it in your wallet and use it to choose the fish you buy. For more details about their recommendations go to www.oceansalive.org/eat.cfm.

When shopping, I avoid the fish on the EPA list, use the Oceans Alive guide, and try to buy local seafood instead of imported seafood and wild-caught fish instead of farm-raised fish. I look for wild-caught fish because some farmed fish (but not all) have been treated with antibiotics and fed pellets contaminated with pesticides. I don't buy the same type of fish each time I shop because eating a variety of fish reduces my exposure to contaminants that might be found in one species. Despite all these concerns, the health benefits of fish are very significant, and I believe the current attention and focus on fish safety is forcing the industry to police itself. I am optimistic that things will only get better, particularly if we consumers choose the types of fish that are proven to be most healthful and safe.

Environmental Defense Best Fish Choices

Abalone (U.S. farmed)
Anchovies
Arctic char (farmed)
Atlantic herring (U.S., Canada)
Catfish (U.S. farmed)
Caviar (U.S. farmed)
Clams (farmed)
Crab (Dungeness, snow [Canada], stone)
Crawfish (U.S.)
Mackerel (Atlantic)
Mahi-mahi (U.S., Atlantic)
Mussels (farmed)
Oysters (farmed)
Pacific halibut (Alaska)
Sablefish/black cod (Alaska)
Salmon, canned pink/sockeye
Salmon, wild (Alaska)
Sardines
Scallops, bay (farmed)
Shrimp (U.S. farmed)
Shrimp, northern (Canada)
Shrimp, Oregon pink
Spot prawns
Striped bass (farmed)
Sturgeon (U.S. farmed)
Tilapia (U.S.)

Preparation. To cook a small piece of fish for your baby, place a fillet of 1–2 ounces in a microwave-safe dish, cover, and cook on high for 60 seconds. Puree until smooth, adding a little water if it appears dry (though you probably won't need much, if any, because fish contains a lot of water). See Baby's First Fish, page 119.

Tip. Fried fish products usually are made from leaner white-fleshed fish. They do not carry the same health benefits as other fish because they tend to have low amounts of the health-promoting omega-3 fatty acids. Also, they may contain trans fatty acids if hydrogenated fat is used in cooking; check the label.

Storage. Use cooked fish within 24 hours or freeze in ice cube trays for up to 1 month.

Caution. Avoid raw fish. Avoid smoked fish cured with nitrates or nitrites.

Family Table. Try Baked Fish* and Fish with Pasta.*

Flaxseed

Flaxseeds look like reddish brown sesame seeds. They carry a lot of fiber and some protein. Flaxseed oil and pure ground flaxseed are not recommended for infants as they can be too rich in fat and the latter too high in fiber. Instead, use ground flaxseed to replace 1 tablespoon of the flour in baked goods. They are a very good source of omega-3 fatty acids.

Grapefruit

Grapefruit is available all year, though it's cheapest January through May, when it is most plentiful. It comes in white or red varieties. Grapefruit is a good source of vitamin C and fiber. Skin discolorations and scratches do not indicate the quality of the fruit, but if the fruit is pointed at the stem end, it is likely to be thick-skinned and have less juice than the thinner-skinned variety.

Preparation. For children twelve months and older, halve grapefruits and remove sections with a knife. Or peel, remove the white pith, and cut between the tough membranes. Serve raw. Canned grapefruit with no sugar added is a good alternative to fresh.

Storage. Grapefruit can last 1–2 weeks if kept refrigerated.

Family Table. Use in fruit salads, or halve and eat for breakfast.

Grapes (buy organic)

Look for organic grapes for your baby, as some grapes are treated with antimicrobial spray. Look for plump grapes, and examine the stems, which should look clean and fresh, not withered. Taste one for sweetness before buying. The most popular are Thompson green seedless and red seedless.

Preparation. Serve chopped grapes when your child is old enough to eat table foods. Grapes are not a recommended baby food because the skins are hard to puree.

Storage. Organic grapes will last about 3 days in the refrigerator.

Caution. Always serve young children grapes sliced in half or in quarters to prevent choking.

Haddock

See Fish.

Ham

See Pork, Ham.

Kasha

See Buckwheat.

Kidney Beans

See Beans, Dried.

Kiwifruit

These egg-size green fruits with fuzzy skin and edible black seeds have an eye-popping color that appeals to many children. The skin is edible if scrubbed, but do not serve it to children because most will not like the texture. They are available year-round and are a great vitamin C source.

Preparation. Cut in half and run a spoon between the skin and the fruit to scoop out the flesh. Chop and serve raw as a finger food to toddlers.

Storage. Select kiwis that are smooth, not shriveled, and not mushy. Ripen kiwis at room temperature in a paper bag.

Caution. Kiwifruit carries the enzyme actinidin, which is used commercially to tenderize meat. This substance also keeps gelatin from setting if raw kiwi is added to it. Though this is not a problem for older children or adults, this natural enzyme might cause a skin irritation in infants, so hold off until your child is on table foods.

Family Table. Serve in fruit salad or to garnish any cold dessert or pudding.

Lamb

Lamb has a strong flavor that many infants like. Often it is the meat used in food allergy elimination diets because it is rarely the cause of a food allergy. Try offering lamb at nine months. It is an excellent source of protein and a good source of iron and zinc. Serve it pureed to infants and chopped as a table food to older children.

Preparation. For cooked lamb, chop into ½-inch pieces. Or sauté 4 ounces ground lamb, drain fat, and press in a paper towel to remove as much fat as possible. To puree, pulse ½ cup cooked meat in a food processor until pasty, then add enough water or vegetable broth (about 2 tablespoons) to make a smooth puree.

Storage. Handle as you would beef (see page 64). Use ground lamb within 2 days of purchase. Freeze leftover puree in ice cube trays and use within 1 month.

Caution. Lamb carries the same risk for cross-contamination as poultry or beef.

Family Table. Serve lamb roasted or grilled, or try Mediterranean Lamb Stew.*

Leeks

A leek looks like a giant scallion. You won't serve it alone as baby food, but it is added to soups and stews for flavor. Use only the white and light green portions. Leeks must be very well washed; sometimes grit and dirt can make its way between the vegetable's layers.

Family Table. Leek Soup.*

Mango

A lovely orange-yellow fruit rich in vitamin C and vitamin A, the mango is native to Southeast Asia and is now grown in Florida and California, among other places. This fruit has a peach-like flavor and creamy texture when ripe.

Preparation. Wash the mango and peel the skin. With a sharp knife cut the mango lengthwise in long strips following the long, skinny, oval-shaped seed that makes up its center. You will then have nice thick strips of juicy fruit that can be pureed, mashed, or chopped and served as a finger food to older children.

Caution. The skin of a mango contains an irritant that might cause contact dermatitis in sensitive people. Avoid contact with the skin, and when you introduce the food, watch for any sensitivities or irritations, especially around the mouth.

Melon

There are many varieties of melon, including cantaloupe (muskmelon), casaba (shaped like a pumpkin), Crenshaw (pale orange flesh), honeydew (white-green skin and green flesh), honeyball (looks like a small honeydew), Persian (looks like a very round cantaloupe), and of course the very popular watermelon. It is very hard to tell how good a melon will be just by looking at it, but the surface should yield just slightly when pressed, and there will be a slight pleasant fruity aroma. Casaba melons do not carry an aroma. All melons are a great source of vitamin C, and the orange variety are a good source of beta-carotene (the vitamin A precursor).

Preparation. Simply slice, cut or scoop the flesh away from the rind, and chop, or slice into wedges. It can also be pureed (though it may need to be strained).

Storage. Keep melon at room temperature until ripe. Refrigerate when ripe or once cut. Can be frozen, but it loses flavor.

Caution. Always wash the rind with soap and water before slicing. It's a good idea for the whole family, not just for babies. Any melon can carry bacteria on its rind, and when it is sliced, the knife can carry the bacteria into the flesh. Washing reduces this risk.

Milk

Do not serve cow's milk until after twelve months, but when you do, buy organic milk or milk from cows not treated with hormones (see page 188). Stick with unflavored milk. Strawberry, chocolate, and vanilla flavors have the same protein and calcium content but an additional 15 grams of carbohydrates, mostly as sugar. Only pasteurized milk should be served to children.

Types of Milk

Dairy Milks

Buttermilk is thick and creamy, tasting more like yogurt than milk. It is low in fat but rich in calcium and protein. Most often used in baking, but it can be drunk.

Evaporated milk is milk that has had 60 percent of the water removed. It is not a substitute for infant formula.

Goat's milk has much less folic acid (1 microgram per 8 ounces) than human milk (16 micrograms) and cow's milk (12 micrograms). Calories and total protein are similar to cow's milk. A child with a cow's milk allergy may also be allergic to goat's milk.

Nonfat dry milk is sold as a powder. All the water has been removed as well as the fat. Usually fortified with vitamins A and D, it can be reconstituted and used by adults for drinking or in baking. On the advice of your baby's doctor, this can be added to formula for infants who are not gaining weight and need an additional source of calories.

Reduced-fat milk comes in fat-free, 1 percent, and 2 percent varieties. It is fortified with vitamin D. Because of its lower fat and calorie content (and sometimes higher protein content, which can be hard for young kidneys to deal with) it is not usually recommended until after age two. Most adults, however, should be drinking skim or 1 percent milk because it provides all the nutrition of whole milk with fewer fat calories.

Sweetened condensed milk is whole milk with added sugar and 50 percent of the water removed. It is used for baking.

Whole milk is what you want to start your baby on at twelve months! Milk fresh from the cow contains fat that rises to the top; homogenization breaks the fat into such small particles that it stays suspended in the milk. It is sold as homogenized milk. Vitamin D is added to ensure adequate nutrition.

Non-Dairy Milks

Almond milk can be used in baking. It contains no cholesterol or lactose, but it is not a substitute for cow's milk because it does not have the same nutrients.

Horchata is made of almonds, rice, or barley. Though it may look "milky," it does not offer the same nutrients as cow's milk.

Rice milk contains more carbohydrates and not as much protein or calcium as cow's milk. Some commercial brands are fortified with calcium, B vitamins, and iron. It can be used as a substitute in baking but it is not a replacement for formula or cow's milk.

Soy milk is usually fortified with calcium but lower in fat than whole cow's milk (about 4 grams per cup). There are 6–7 grams protein and only 80 calories per 8 ounces, too few calories for babies and most young children.

Millet

An ancient grain native to Africa and Asia, millet was mostly sold as birdseed in the United States until recently. Millet is now finding its way to our table as cereal or a side dish. It has a very high protein content for a grain. The grains are very small yellow pellets.

Preparation. Combine ¼ cup millet with ¾ cup water, bring to a boil, reduce heat, cover, and simmer until tender, at least 20 minutes. Serve this when your child is ready for a new texture. The cooked grain is lumpy.

Storage. Like all grains, millet will last a long time in a cool, dark, dry location.

Family Table. Before boiling, toast the grains to bring out the flavor. Put the amount of grain you want to cook in a pan and heat until the grain browns slightly. Stir constantly to prevent burning. Add three parts water to each part grain and a little butter or oil to prevent sticking.

Mushrooms

The white button mushroom is the most widely available. Mushrooms supply some B vitamins, minerals, and antioxidants, but are not a rich source of nutrients and for that reason are not encouraged as a baby food. Criminis, portabellos, and shiitakes can be used interchangeably in recipes, but they do not carry more nutrients. Do use them to add flavor to stews and soups when your child is older. Look for mushrooms that have a smooth, creamy cap. Avoid those with a pitted surface or dark discolorations. Most mushrooms are grown on commercial farms in controlled sterile environments.

Storage. Keep fresh mushrooms refrigerated for up to 1 week.

Family Table. Use in salad, stuff with vegetables as an appetizer, and use in casseroles, stews, and sautés.

Nectarine (buy organic)

See Peaches.

Noodles

See Pasta.

Nuts

Eventually nuts should be part of your child's diet, as research shows us that people who regularly eat nuts tend to have healthier hearts. If there is a history of nut allergy in your family, however, do not add nuts until after the first birthday and possibly even longer. Nuts are one of the top four allergens, and when eaten by a child susceptible to a nut allergy early in life, they can lead to a lifelong allergy. Ask your baby's doctor for advice on this issue. Read more about food allergies on page 17.

Once you do add nuts, nut butters, such as peanut butter and al-mond butter can be a delicious protein source. Use nut butters in sandwiches, as a dip with vegetables, or mixed with a little broth and used as a topping on pasta.

Caution. All nuts pose a potential choking risk, so avoid these until your child has teeth and is chewing real food.

Family Table. The most healthful nuts, according to the Food and Drug Administration, include almonds, hazelnuts, peanuts (techni-cally a legume), pecans, pignoli (pine nuts), pistachios, and wal-nuts. Sprinkle nuts on salad instead of cheese, use nut butters in sandwiches, and serve peanut sauce or nut-based pesto instead of a meat- or cheese-based sauce on pasta.

Oatmeal

The oatmeal that most of us buy has been steamed and rolled flat. Quick-cooking oats have been cut into smaller pieces to reduce cooking time. Instant oats have been precooked and dried before being rolled. Steel-cut oats, also called Irish oatmeal, have not been steamed and rolled but rather are chopped with blades and look coarse and granular compared to the others. Steel-cut oats take longer to cook and often benefit from being soaked overnight. Most children will prefer rolled oats over steel-cut oats. Oats are a good source of soluble fiber, the type of fiber that helps keep cho-lesterol levels low.

Serve infant oatmeal to your baby because it has no sugar added and is fortified with iron. Rolled and steel-cut oats do not have added iron. When your child is older, be very careful about your oatmeal choices. Avoid sweetened instant oatmeal products, many of which contain high-fructose corn syrup. It is better to make your own plain oatmeal and blend with fruit, honey, or even sugar.

Olive Oil

See Cooking Oils and Other Dietary Fats.

Onions

Onions are not a baby food, but they can be part of meals for older children because they add flavor. They are available in red, yellow, or white varieties, have very few calories, and supply small amounts of a variety of nutrients.

Preparation. Long cooking gives onions a delicious sweet taste. Slice 2 medium white or yellow onions (about 1 cup) and place in a medium saucepan with 2 tablespoons olive oil. Cover and cook over low heat for 10 minutes, stirring often, until the onion is soft. Remove the cover and continue cooking for another 10 minutes. The onions are done when they are golden. If they look dry or start to burn, add a little water. Chop and mix to taste with cooked meats.

Tip. When you slice into an onion, it releases a natural sulfur compound that causes eyes to tear. There are lots of suggestions for reducing this unpleasant side effect. The best ideas include cutting with a very sharp knife, cutting under running water, and refrigerating for a few minutes before cutting. The best way to remove onion odor from hands is to rub hands with lemon juice.

Family Table. Onions can be added to salads, stews, soups, and pasta dishes.

Oranges

Navel and Valencia are the most popular varieties of oranges. Navel oranges have no seeds, but the Valencias are easier to peel. Oranges should be heavy for their size and not spongy. They are a superb source of vitamin C; one medium orange or 4 ounces orange juice supplies all the vitamin C a child needs daily during the first year.

Preparation. Peel and section. Serve raw when your child is old enough to eat table food.

Family Table. Serve as a snack, in fruit salad, or as juice (6 ounces of juice per day is a suggested limit).

Papaya

Available year-round, most of it coming from Hawaii, the flesh of papaya has a rich orange color that indicates it is a good source of vitamin A. It also supplies vitamin C and fiber. Look for fruit that feels soft but not mushy to the touch. The skin of papayas turns from green to yellow-orange as the fruit ripens. Papaya contains a natural chemical called papain, used to tenderize meat. The amount diminishes with ripening. The center of a papaya is filled with shiny black seeds that can be dried, ground, and used as a substitute for black pepper, but are not to be served to babies.

Preparation. Wash the skin, slice in half, remove the tiny black seeds and discard, and scoop out the flesh. It can be pureed; no added water is needed. Serve plain or mix with yogurt or cereal.

Storage. Can be frozen in chunks in a plastic bag or pureed and frozen in an ice cube tray. A papaya can last in the refrigerator for 7–10 days depending on ripeness.

Family Table. Papaya can be used in fruit salads or sliced and eaten as a snack. Try folding it into cold puddings for a tangy addition.

Parsnips

Buy these in late winter when their flavor is the sweetest. They look like a pale carrot but have a delicious taste your kids are likely to enjoy. Mashing or pureeing seems to enhance their flavor. Buy small parsnips, because the larger ones have a coarse woody center that will need to be removed.

Preparation. Peel and chop into ½-inch pieces. Cover with water, bring to a boil, reduce heat, and simmer, covered, for 4–8 minutes or until tender when pierced with a fork. You can also cook them in the microwave on high for 1½ minutes. Allow to cool, and drain, reserving liquid. Puree with enough cooking water to make it smooth and fluffy. For older children, mash with a little cooking liquid. Parsnips are particularly delicious when blended with fruit such as banana, pears, or plums.

Storage. Keep refrigerated and use within 2 weeks. Cooked pureed parsnips can be frozen in an ice cube tray and used within 1 month.

Family Table. Boil and mash with butter, salt, and pepper. Or slice into even-size pieces, toss with a little olive oil, salt, and pepper, and roast until tender (about 20 minutes at 375°F). Turn at least once while cooking.

Pasta

Most children and babies love pasta, and there is a shape and size for everyone. When my children were little, the small rice-shaped pasta called orzo was our favorite. Now we eat more whole-grain pasta and experiment with Asian rice noodles and wheat udon noodles. For babies, offer whole-grain or enriched pasta at around nine months. Follow preparation instructions on the package.

Colored noodles have small amounts of vegetables added, but this adds very little in the way of extra nutrition. Be cautious of ramen noodles because they are steamed, fried, and air-dried before packaging and carry a great deal more fat and sodium than most other noodles.

Peaches (buy organic)

Peaches and their smooth-skinned relatives nectarines come in white- or yellow-fleshed varieties. They can ripen and develop flavor after picking, but they can be mealy if they are stored at too cold a temperature—something you may not know until you bite into one. Locally grown varieties will taste the best. Peaches are a good source of fiber and vitamins.

Preparation. Peel, pit, and chop. Peaches can also be pureed with a little juice. You can microwave chopped peaches for 1 minute before mashing or pureeing. To make peeling easier, dip into boiling water for 1 minute, then run under cold water and peel.

Storage. Once ripe, peaches will keep in the refrigerator for 5–7 days. Fruit cut in half and pitted can be frozen.

Tip. Peaches are classified as freestone (the flesh easily separates from the pit) or clingstone (the flesh sticks to the pit). Clingstone peaches are the varieties most often canned.

Family Table. Peaches are delicious eaten out of hand, but also try them in Free-form Fruit Tart* or use to replace apples in a crisp* or as the fruit in Fruit Cobbler* or to replace berries in Blueberry Muffins.*

Peanuts, Peanut Butter

See Nuts.

Pears (buy organic)

Pears come in several varieties (Bartlett is the most popular) and are delicious; their flavor is most pronounced at room temperature. They are a good source of fiber and vitamins A and C as well as potassium. Look for firm fruit with smooth skin. Hard pears can ripen at room temperature. Choose those that already feel a little soft—this increases the chances the fruit will ripen as desired. Don't ripen in plastic because they are sensitive to the carbon dioxide that accumulates.

Preparation. Do not peel; the skins are so thin that they almost disappear when pureed. They can also be removed by straining if desired. Scrub, slice in half, and remove the core and seeds. To cook, place cut side down on a plate and microwave for 1 minute or until tender. Cool and drain, reserving the liquid, then cut into chunks and puree or mash, adding the reserved cooking liquid as needed.

Family Table. Serve poached*, or in a tart* or cobbler*.

Peas, Fresh

Green peas are what we think of most at the mention of the word "peas," but snow peas with their edible pods and sugar snaps are also favorite finger foods for toddlers. Infants will like the conventional round peas best. Buy peas in the pod and shell, or buy frozen peas. Avoid canned peas, as most have a high sodium content. Peas carry more protein than most vegetables and they are a good source of fiber.

Preparation. Measure ½ cup fresh or frozen peas (if fresh remove from pod first). One pound of peas in the pod will yield about 1 cup of edible peas. Add peas and 2 tablespoons water to a saucepan, cover, and boil until tender, about 5–6 minutes. Or place in a steamer and steam until tender, also 5–6 minutes. Microwave ½ cup peas with 1 tablespoon water for 3 minutes, covered, then let rest for 1 minute. Puree peas with enough cooking liquid to reach desired consistency, or mash with a fork. When serving to a toddler, mash the peas a little so they roll less and are easier for a young child to master when learning to eat with utensils.

Storage. Fresh peas won't keep long, so use them quickly. Peas can keep at most 3–4 days refrigerated in a plastic bag, but don't remove the shell until ready to cook.

Family Table. Steam or boil fresh or frozen peas.

Peppers (buy organic)

Sweet bell peppers carry none of the fiery ingredient, capsaicin, found in chile peppers. Red peppers are the sweetest, but green peppers are most plentiful. Orange, yellow, purple, brown, and even white peppers are also available. Look for peppers with deep color. They should feel heavy for their size and their walls should be firm. Soft spots indicate decay. All peppers are an excellent source of vitamin C.

Preparation. For older children, grate any color pepper, cut into thin strips, or chop. This is a favorite dipping vegetable. Cooked pureed red peppers can make an appealing sauce. Bring a pot of water to a boil. Slice a large pepper in half, remove seeds and white ribs, add to boiling water, and cook for 5 minutes. Remove and put in an ice water bath until the pieces are cold. This loosens the skin. Rub the skin with your finger; it should come off in big strips. Squeeze out excess water and puree the pepper until smooth. The sauce will be thin. Serve over rice or noodles in small amounts or mix with other meats and grains.

Storage. Peppers can last 5–7 days depending on age. Keep refrigerated.

Caution. Unlike bell peppers, chile peppers contain capsaicin, a spicy substance that can cause severe irritation. Though chile peppers are part of the diet of many cultures and young people learn to love them, they are not to be served to infants. Be cautious when preparing chile peppers in your own kitchen. They should not come in contact with baby food. When preparing fiery peppers, wear gloves so the irritating oils will not transfer from your skin to your baby's.

Black or white pepper, a spice from a berry that grows on vines, is not related to bell or chile peppers. These have no place in your baby's diet, either.

Family Table. Bell peppers can be used raw in salad or cooked, as in Stuffed Peppers.* Chile peppers and ground black or white pepper are great ways to add flavor to adult's and older children's meals without adding sodium.

Persimmons

This yellow-orange fruit is native to China and was introduced to California in the 1800s. There are two kinds of persimmons. Hachiya persimmons must be allowed to ripen until very soft or else they will be extremely astringent. Fuyu persimmons are firm when ripe.

Preparation. For Hachiyas, cut in half and scoop out pulp with a spoon. Fuyus can be eaten out of hand.

Storage. Refrigerate once ripe.

Family Table. Fuyus can be used in a tart or fruit salad like an apple or pear; the Hachiya is almost always used as a puree in breads, cakes, puddings, or sauces.

Pineapple

These large prickly fruits are available year-round, but prices are best in late spring, when they are most abundant. A ripe pineapple has more yellow than green and a pleasant sweet aroma. Choose the largest pineapples you can, as they will have a greater proportion of edible fruit. Pineapple will ripen at room temperature within a few days.

Preparation. Slice the top off the pineapple. With a sharp knife cut off the skin in long lengthwise strips. Cut out any hard eyes that remain. Cut in half, then quarters. Cut off the point of each quarter to remove the hard center core, then cut into chunks. Pineapple is best served raw as a finger food or in bite-size pieces to older children. It is not usually recommended for infants under six months because it is so fibrous. However, a ripe sweet pineapple can be pureed and blended with cereal or yogurt for a flavorful treat.

Tip. Frozen pineapple is an easy and nutritious treat. Dole brand has cubes that have no sugar added and can be ready for eating after thawing for just 20 minutes. Canned pineapple in water or juice is also a convenient and economical source.

Storage. Once ripe, store in the refrigerator. Use within 3–5 days.

Family Table. Pineapples are fabulous between meals as a snack or as a part of a fruit salad. They are also great in the classic upside-down cake or in muffins.

Plums

Plums come in a variety of shapes and sizes. The flavor and sweetness vary with each variety; I usually prefer the large purple plum with dark flesh. Fresh plums should feel soft but firm. Dried plums, also known as prunes, are a good source of fiber and vitamin C, and a great way to satisfy a sweet tooth. Pureed fresh plums are a delicious addition to cooked grains, and stewed dried prunes blend nicely with cooked meat.

Preparation. Cut fresh plums in half, remove the pit, and chop. Put ½ cup chopped plum in a saucepan, add 1 tablespoon juice or water, cover, and simmer for 3–4 minutes, or microwave for 1 minute. Puree with the skins still on (the skin is thin and disappears once pureed). You may not need to add any of the cooking liquid depending on the fruit. For dried plums, pour ¼ cup boiling water over ½ cup dried fruit and let stew until mushy, about 10 minutes.

Puree for infants or mash with a fork for older kids. Add juice if needed to thin it out.

Storage. Dried plums can last 4–6 weeks if kept in an airtight container in a cool dark spot. Fresh plums can be ripened at room temperature; store ripe fruit in the refrigerator.

Caution. Prunes act as a laxative, probably because they are a natural source of sorbitol, which is not well digested and causes frequent bowel movements. This is a great tool for treating constipation but an obvious problem if you're traveling and diaper changing is difficult.

Family Table. Use plum puree to top ice cream or frozen yogurt, or use plums in Free-form Fruit Tart.*

Pork, Ham

Today's pork is much leaner than it was a century ago and as a result more popular. Ham is pork that has been cured with salt to prevent spoilage, though today the process is used more for flavor than as a preservative. Look for well-trimmed meat that is pink and not gray; chops and the pork loin are the leanest cuts. Ham will contain about 400 mg sodium per ounce; fresh pork 20 mg sodium per ounce.

Preparation. Chop well-cooked pork and puree or finely chop depending on age. Do not serve ham to very young children because of its high sodium content.

Storage. Fresh pork can last 2–4 days if wrapped in plastic and refrigerated.

Caution. Better production methods have reduced the fear of food poisoning from undercooked pork; however, it is still to be cooked to an internal temperature of 160°F. Read preparation instructions carefully as not all ham is fully cooked.

Family Table. Pork Tenderloin*

Potatoes (buy organic)

All varieties of white-, yellow-, or purple-fleshed potatoes have a similar nutrition profile. They have a little protein, some potassium and fiber, and small amounts of B vitamins, calcium, and vitamin C.

They are naturally low in sodium. Unfortunately, most of the potatoes fed to children are in the form of french fries and potato chips, foods that are excessive in sodium and total fat. I personally love Yukon gold for making the creamiest mashed potatoes; russets are my favorite for baking, and I prefer red new potatoes for steaming. If you are lucky, your market will carry fingerling potatoes and even purple potatoes. These are heirloom vegetables being resurrected to diversify the food supply.

Preparation. To mash, peel potatoes and cut into equal-size pieces. Place in a sauce pan, cover with water, and bring to a boil, then reduce heat and simmer until tender, about 5–8 minutes. Use a fork to test for doneness. Drain and mash with a little breast milk, formula, or juice for younger babies, with milk and a little butter for older babies. Do not add salt for babies and young children.

To bake, wash the potato, prick the skin, and bake at 350°F until tender, about 35–45 minutes depending on size. If you insert a metal skewer before baking, it will cook in half the time. Chop, or mash as previously described. To microwave, wash the potato, prick the skin, and microwave for 2 minutes, then let rest for 1 minute. Cook longer if it is not soft to the touch. Chop or mash.

Storage. Potatoes can last for months in a cool dark spot.

Caution. The green color sometimes seen on potatoes is caused by exposure to light and indicates the presence of a natural but potentially harmful chemical called solanine. A small adult would have to eat 2 cups of entirely green potatoes to become ill, but since infants and toddlers are so small, even lesser amounts could cause problems. For them, avoid potatoes with green patches.

Prunes

See Plums.

Quinoa

Pronounced "keen-wa," quinoa is a tiny, flavorful soft grain from South America. It comes in a variety of colors, from a light cream color to almost black. Quinoa has a very high protein content for a grain—½ cup dry quinoa has 11 grams of protein, while an equal amount of rice has only 5 grams.

Preparation. Rinse 1 cup of quinoa in cold water and drain. Bring 2 cups of water to a boil, stir in the quinoa, and add 1 teaspoon cooking oil. Cover, reduce heat, and simmer for 20 minutes, until tender.

Tip. Most quinoa is washed before being sold to remove the natural bitter-tasting coating called saponin. I suggest rinsing for babies just in case.

Family Table. Serve instead of rice or pasta for a change of pace. Try toasting the dry grain before cooking, which gives it a deeper flavor.

Radishes

Radishes are not recommended as a baby food because they are bitter and not very nutritious, with few calories and only a little bit of fiber. Toddlers eighteen months and older will like their color and might enjoy them as part of a vegetable plate. Choose radishes less than 1 inch in diameter with good bright color and plump round shape. Avoid radishes with decayed tops.

Preparation. Rinse and slice into strips or grate.

Caution. Because radishes are hard and round, they can pose a risk for choking. Do not serve whole or cut into coin shapes.

Family Table. Radishes are a good no-calorie snack that adds crunch and sharp flavor to salads.

Raisins

Raisins are not an infant food but they will make a nice snack for toddlers. Raisins, of course, are dried grapes. They contain fiber and they also have some iron, calcium, and potassium. Look for unsulfured raisins.

Raspberries

When choosing raspberries (and blackberries), select firm, plump berries with no signs of mold. Toddlers can eat raw berries; for younger babies, cook and strain to remove seeds.

Preparation. Rinse right before using.

To cook, place ½ cup berries in a saucepan, add 1 tablespoon water, bring to a boil, then reduce heat and simmer for 2 minutes. Let cool, then strain to remove seeds. Mix with yogurt or other cooked fruit.

Storage. Use fresh berries within a day.

Family Table. Mix berries into fruit salad, bake in a Free-form Fruit Tart,* or substitute for blueberries in Blueberry Muffins.*

Rhubarb

This is food for the family table but not your baby's plate. To make it palatable you must cook it slowly with a lot of sugar. It has been nicknamed America's pie plant because we use it almost exclusively to make pie. It is an excellent source of calcium (about 100 milligrams in 4 ounces), but it is also rich in oxalic acid, which binds with the calcium to make it unabsorbable. In fact, the leaves are so rich in oxalic acid they can be harmful to pets and little ones. Fortunately, their bitter taste makes them unappealing. Look for stems that are glossy in color. Usually the smaller thin stalks are the most tender. Discard the leaves.

Family Table. Use in pies or to make Free-form Fruit Tart.*

Rice

In many cultures rice is a staple of life. There are dozens of varieties of rice to choose from: jasmine, Texmati, and wild pecan (all aromatic), basmati (a slender, long grain), glutinous (used in Asian cooking, it has a sticky quality), arborio (used for making risotto), wehani (dark-colored). Wild rice is actually not a rice at all but a grass.

Most of the varieties listed above will not be sold as whole grains—they usually have the bran removed, making cooking time shorter and the grain more tender but lowering fiber content and some nutrients. However, that processing can also make them more digestible (read about phytic acid on page 222). Choose rice that fits your recipes, cooking style, and taste buds. Brown rice is my favorite whole-grain rice.

Preparation. For white rice, bring 1 cup of water to a boil, add ½ cup rice, cover, reduce heat to low, and cook 20 minutes, until tender. For brown rice, use ½ cup rice to 1 cup plus 2 tablespoons water and cook for 45 minutes. For other varieties, refer to package instructions.

Tip. I used to turn up my nose at instant products, but instant rices have gotten better. I always keep Uncle Ben's Ready Rice brown rice in my cupboard, as it can be ready in 90 seconds in the microwave.

Rice Milk

See Milk.

Salmon

See Fish.

Soybeans

The soybean is an ancient food and a source of protein for many cultures. Fresh soybeans (edamame) can be boiled and eaten as a vegetable, pressed to make soybean oil, turned into soybean curd (*see* Tofu), or fermented to make soy sauce and tempeh. They can be dried and turned into soy flour, used as the protein source in textured vegetable protein (TVP), and of course used to make soy milk and soy-based infant formula.

However, there is a heated controversy over whether there are health risks associated with soy. Soybeans contain the isoflavones genistein, daidzin, and glycitin, which are phytoestrogens. In large doses (such as in supplements) isolated isoflavones have been linked with health problems in animals. Also, soybeans naturally have a high concentration of phytic acid, which binds to minerals and blocks the absorption of calcium, magnesium, iron, and especially zinc (read about phytic acid on page 222). Finally, almost all the soybeans now in production are genetically modified. Because of these concerns, I do not recommend soy supplements, but I do encourage the use of soy foods as part of a varied diet. I like soy foods because they have been part of the human diet for centuries, they taste good, and they are a plant-based source of protein with no saturated fat.

In regard to soy formula, the American Academy of Pediatrics recommends the use of soy formula as an alternative to cow's-milk-based formula only for infants unable to tolerate cow's milk due to allergy or lactase deficiency, and for those families wanting a vegetarian diet for their child. Soy formula is not advised for preterm infants, or for the prevention of colic or prevention of allergies.

Preparation. Edamame can be found in the frozen food case. They can be used in soups or salads, or served as a vegetable like peas.

Caution. Soy sauce is not to be served to infants because it contains more than 1,000 milligrams of sodium per tablespoon, an amount excessive for a young child.

Spaghetti Squash

See Zucchini.

Spinach (buy organic)

Spinach is a good source of iron, potassium, vitamin A, riboflavin, and vitamin C. It is also a good source of calcium, but the natural oxalate in spinach binds with the calcium, making it less available to the body. Look for leaves that are crisp and tender with small stems.

Preparation. Pick over leaves and discard any that look withered. Rinse spinach very well because sand can cling to its broad leaves. Much bagged spinach is triple-washed already, but I prefer to rinse all my vegetables just to be sure. Frozen spinach is an easy alternative to fresh.

Preparation. Steam 10 ounces of fresh spinach for 3 minutes, stir to redistribute the leaves, then steam 2 minutes more. Or bring 1 quart water to a boil, add 1 pound spinach, reduce heat, and simmer 3–4 minutes. Cool slightly, then squeeze out excess water. Puree until very smooth; extra liquid will probably not be needed.

Storage. Fresh spinach should be washed, stored in a plastic bag, and used within 2 days. Freeze puree in ice cube trays.

Caution. In 2006 an outbreak of illness from *E. coli* in organic spinach killed three people, one of them a young child. Many were surprised that *E. coli* could be present in organic foods, but organic produce that is grown in dirt can come into contact with animal manure, a source of *E. coli*. In most cases washing and cooking will take care of any microbes. Since children are particularly vulnerable, it is recommended that spinach be cooked before being served to a child.

Family Table. Spinach is delicious steamed or sauteed and tossed with a little balsamic vinegar.

Squash, Summer

See Zucchini.

Squash, Winter

Acorn and butternut seem to be the most popular members of the winter squash family, but there are other equally delicious varieties, including buttercup, Hubbard (blue and green), delicata, and banana. A good squash should have a hard tough skin and it should feel heavy for its size. Squash is a superb source of vitamin A and fiber, and it is a vegetable that many infants and children love.

Preparation. Cut squash in half, scoop out seeds, and bake at 350°F for at least 60 minutes, until tender. It can also be microwaved to save time. Place the squash cut side down and microwave for 7–8 minutes. To puree, scoop out flesh and discard skin; puree with a little water, broth, or juice.

Storage. Freeze leftover puree in ice cube trays and use within 1 month.

Family Table. Serve squash baked, steamed, or cut into chunks and roasted. Mash cooked squash with butter, salt, and pepper to taste, or try mashing with maple syrup and add cinnamon or freshly grated nutmeg.

Strawberries (buy organic)

Strawberries are most abundant in late spring and early summer but are now grown year-round. Children eight months and up love them. Avoid berries with large pale areas, as they are likely to be flavorless, and check the box for mold, particularly toward the bottom of the package, as it can spread quickly, ruining the berries before you can enjoy them. Instead of buying flavorless strawberries out of season, try frozen unsweetened berries. These are not as good as fresh, but they can be added to muffin or pancake batter and used to make fruit smoothies.

Preparation. Trim tops and chop.

Family Table. Serve in fruit salads, Berry Pancakes,* or Free-form Fruit Tart.*

Sweet Potato

Sweet potatoes have yellow or orange flesh; the skin can be white, yellow, red, orange, or purple. Look for sweet potatoes that have a clean, smooth skin, with no marks of decay. They are a great source of potassium, fiber, and vitamin A. Sometimes sweet potatoes are called yams, but the true yam is a starchy tropical tuber and is not grown commercially in the United States.

Preparation. Scrub, prick the skin, and bake at 350°F for 60 minutes or until very soft. Or scrub, prick, and microwave for 3 minutes, or until soft. Alternatively, peel, cut into ½-inch chunks, cover with water, and boil until tender. Mash cooked sweet potato, or puree with a little liquid. Freeze in ice cube trays and keep for 1 month.

Tip. A 4-ounce sweet potato has a little more calcium and fiber than a white potato, and a lot more vitamin A. The best thing about sweet potatoes is that we usually eat them in a healthful manner, while white potatoes often end up topped with sour cream, fried, or turned into chips.

Storage. Do not refrigerate raw sweet potatoes; store in a cool, dark spot. Freeze cooked puree in an ice cube tray for up to 1 month.

Tempeh

Tempeh is fermented soybeans pressed into cakes. Available in many health food stores and some supermarkets, it has a mild flavor and a firm texture. A 6-ounce portion provides 32 grams of protein, making it a good source of plant-based protein.

Preparation. Tempeh is precooked. It can be served mashed by itself or with other foods such as pureed vegetables. It can also be chopped and served as a finger food.

Tofu

Tofu is soybean curd. It is a great source of protein and many babies love it, probably because of its smooth texture and bland flavor. Introduce it around nine months.

Tofu can be served in place of meat, fish, poultry, or egg at a meal. It does not need to be cooked. Serve it mashed by itself or mash it with fruit or cooked vegetables. It will make a great finger food when your child is older. When my daughters were around fifteen months I introduced them to tofu hot dogs instead of conventional hot dogs, and they were a hit.

Storage. Tofu is a perishable item. Buy tofu that is individually packaged, carrying a sell-by date for freshness. Keep it covered and refrigerated.

Family Table. Add tofu to salads, stir-fries, or soup.

Tomatoes

Tomatoes ripen best on the vine, and so the most flavorful ones are locally grown. They are a great source of vitamin C and most kids like them when they are older. Tomatoes are not usually a baby food because the seeds and skins need to be removed; also, tomatoes are naturally high in acidity and may cause skin irritations or stomach upsets in young babies. Save tomatoes for children ten months and older. Tomatoes are a great source of vitamin C, and they carry a substance called lycopene that has health benefits including maintaining good vision and cancer prevention. Look for tomatoes that are smooth and deep in color.

Preparation. Chop or slice for children eating finger foods or peel, seed, cook, and puree.

Tip. Commercial tomato products can be a big source of sodium. A medium-size tomato has about 11 milligrams of sodium, but 4 ounces of many brands of tomato juice has 400 milligrams sodium, and 4 ounces of tomato sauce can have 740 milligrams sodium. Use fresh tomatoes or no-salt-added products.

Storage. Tomatoes can be kept at room temperature. Do not refrigerate tomatoes, because it makes the tomato lose flavor and become watery.

Tuna

See Fish.

Turkey

Turkey isn't just for Thanksgiving. Ground turkey is a good alternative to beef, because it is lower in fat and calories. The dark meat of turkey is a particularly rich source of zinc.

Preparation. Puree ¼ cup chopped cooked turkey until it is pasty, then add enough water or broth until puree is smooth; or simply chop cooked turkey and mix with vegetables for older children. Form ground turkey into small patties, cook and serve as you would ground beef. Puree for young children; chop for toddlers.

Caution. Always avoid cross-contamination of poultry products with food that will not be cooked, as well as countertops and utensils. Be sure to cook thoroughly.

Storage. Ground turkey spoils faster than whole turkey or turkey pieces.

Family Table. Try Meatballs* and Hamburger Soup* made with ground turkey.

Turnip

Turnips are a root vegetable with a whitish bottom and purple top. They are sometimes sold with the greens attached, like carrots. A good source of fiber and potassium, turnips have a strong flavor and taste best when mashed or pureed; you can mix turnips with mashed potato or other vegetable. They have a thick skin that must be peeled before cooking. Look for turnips that are firm and small to medium in size.

Rutabagas are in the turnip family but are yellow fleshed and usually bigger than turnips. They are often sold with a wax coating on the skin to preserve freshness. They are cooked in the same way as turnips but may take a few more minutes of cooking time.

Preparation. Peel and chop into ½-inch pieces. Steam for 12–15 minutes or until tender. Extra water will probably not be required for pureeing, but use water or juice if needed. Older children can enjoy them mashed with a little butter and a small amount of milk.

Family Table. Steam and mash with butter and milk. Use salt and pepper to taste.

Walnuts

See Nuts.

Water

Infants rarely need extra water because it comes naturally in breast milk and is in infant formula, but many of you will wonder what type of water will be best once your child does start to drink it, or you may be concerned about it now if you use it to mix formula. Many parents choose to buy bottled water because of the perception that it is safer and purer than tap water, but 25 percent of all bottled water is actually just bottled tap water. The Environmental Protection Agency (EPA) sets standards for tap water in the United States, and in general it is very safe. Bottled water is not without its concerns, either. It is estimated that it takes twenty million barrels of oil each year to make the bottles that carry bottled water, and 90 percent of those bottles are not even recycled. If you want to avoid bottled water but are concerned about potential contaminants in tap water, put your mind at ease and add an NSF-certified water filter. Go to www.nsf.org or www.consumersearch.com/www/kitchen/water-filters/review.html for more information about selecting a water filter for your home.

As an adult, you want water to be your preferred drink, and you want your child to see you drinking water instead of sweetened drinks. Most Americans are consuming more calories and gaining weight in part because of the beverages they choose. Water is the best drink to quench thirst and meet fluid needs. Vitamin-fortified water carries added nutrients, but fortified water is no replacement for food, and it may pose a health risk if too much of one nutrient is consumed; it is never advised for young children or for mixing with formula.

Watermelon

See Melon.

Wax Beans

See Beans, Green and Yellow.

Whole Grains

See Barley, Bread, Buckwheat, Bulgur, Corn, Millet, Oatmeal, Quinoa, Rice

In 2005 the U.S. Dietary Guidelines were revised to clearly state the importance of whole grains in our diet. Consuming whole grains can reduce the risk of chronic disease. The general recommendation for adults is to include at least three servings (an adult serving is 1 slice of bread or ½ cup cooked rice, pasta, or cereal) of whole grains per day. There is no recommendation for infants, but this is a good time to get them started. At two years, the guidelines suggest children eat a slice and a half of whole-grain bread or the equivalent daily to get the health benefits they provide. I recommend that families try to serve whole grains at two out of three meals per day. When shopping for whole-grain products, choose ones that are fortified with the B vitamin folate. It will be clearly stated on the label. Read about whole grains and phytic acid on page 222. See the whole-grain stamp on page 56.

Yam

See Sweet Potato.

Yogurt

Yogurt is a wonderful source of calcium and protein and it can be added to a baby's menu at nine to twelve months as long as it does not replace formula or breast milk, which carry iron. Liquid cow's milk is a poor source of iron, which is the reason you don't use it until after twelve months. Of course, it will need to be avoided if a baby has a cow's milk allergy. Individuals with lactose intolerance can often take yogurt in small amounts, usually 4–8 ounces at a time. Read about lactose intolerance on page 233. Look for yogurt with active cultures, and buy plain whole-milk yogurt for babies.

Preparation. Blend with pureed fruits, vegetables, or grains.

Family Table. Low-fat yogurt that is low in added sugar is an excellent snack and dessert.

Zucchini

Abundant in summer gardens, the summer squashes—zucchini, spaghetti squash, and yellow squash—are mild-flavored vegetables that provide lots of fiber and potassium. For zucchini or yellow squash, choose smaller squash that have a glossy skin; giant squash are likely to be overly mature. Though the seeds are very moist and soft, I don't recommend them for babies; you will have to cook the squash, then strain it. Spaghetti squashes are larger; choose the yellowest.

Preparation. For zucchini and yellow squash, trim the ends but don't peel, and cut into chunks. Put 1 cup of squash in a saucepan with 1 tablespoon water, cover, and cook for 3–4 minutes, until tender. Or steam for 3–5 minutes until tender. Puree the entire cooked vegetable, then strain for young babies; for older children, well-cooked squash will not need to be pureed.

For spaghetti squash, cut squash in half, scoop out the seeds, and place cut side down in a glass baking dish. Add ½ cup water to the dish and bake, covered, for 30 minutes or microwave for 10 minutes, until tender. Scoop out the cooked squash, which will come apart in long strands like spaghetti. Small portions of spaghetti squash can be pureed for babies, and the remainder served at the family table.

Family Table. Toss cooked zucchini, yellow, or spaghetti squash with olive oil and pepper or serve with a little butter or cheese. Zucchini and yellow squash taste delicious when grated raw into a lettuce and tomato salad. Also try Zucchini Muffins.*

FIVE

High Chair Cuisine

There is only a very short period of time when your baby will need food that is truly "baby food." By his first birthday he can eat chopped table foods and finger foods, and by eighteen months he will be curious about what you are having and can eat many family meals. Homemade baby food tastes best because of the freshness of the ingredients. For example, carrots from a jar will taste different from the ones you cook and puree yourself because a jarred version could be on the store shelf for months and flavor will suffer. Besides freshness and flavor, homemade baby food is much less expensive than the jarred kind.

FOOD SAFETY

Food safety can be very simple. Keep things very clean and at the right temperature. Food can cool at room temperature before serving, but discard any food allowed to sit at room temperature for more than 1 hour. In general, when your child is under eight months you must cook most of his food. Banana and avocado do not need to be cooked.

To keep your food safe, always wash hands, keep countertops and food preparation areas clean, and wash fruits and vegetables under running water for at least 30 seconds. Wash fruits with skin even if you plan to peel them, since germs clinging to the skin can be transferred to the fruit when a knife slices through it; washing the skin before slicing, even when it is not to be eaten, will eliminate this risk. Even organic and natural foods can be sources of food-borne illness. The words "organic" and "natural" apply to growing practices, not food safety.

Keep raw, cooked, and ready-to-eat foods separate. Infants and young children are particularly vulnerable to food-borne illness and should not drink raw (unpasteurized) milk or raw or undercooked meat, poultry, fish, or shellfish. Young children should avoid unpasteurized juices and raw sprouts.

To avoid food contamination, follow this simple advice:

- Keep hot food hot and cold food cold.
- Don't feed your baby from the jar food is stored in. Germs will travel from the mouth to the food via the spoon and will potentially cause the food to spoil.
- Buy a food thermometer and use it to measure the temperature of cooked meats.

Go to www.fightbac.org, a great Web site for more practical advice on food safety.

HOW TO PUREE

Pureeing food hardly needs any description, but there are some tips that can make it more successful. First, get the right equipment. Food processors are perfect for making baby food—and also for making breadcrumbs, grinding nuts, and making pesto. There are mini food processors that are easy to clean and store. Several mothers have told me they relied on their blender, which can work well, though I find small amounts of food tend to get stuck under the blade. Another mom told me she received a handheld immersion blender as a gift and loved it. A portable hand-operated food mill can be useful both at home and when traveling, and can be found in stores selling baby and child items.

In general, puree food that is cold or at least allow it to cool to a temperature safe enough to work with. Put the food in first and grind it until it is reduced to chunks or lumps, then add a small amount of liquid. Use cooking liquid, breast milk, formula, Baby Broth (recipe on page 131), or pure unsweetened juice as the added liquid; avoid cow's milk until age one and yogurt until about nine months. How much liquid you add will depend on the food and how smooth you want the puree to be. Well-cooked carrots, well-cooked beets, avocado, and cooked spinach puree easily, as do fruits such as plums, peaches, fresh apricots, and pears. Purchase a small spatula, which can be very useful to scrape down the sides of blenders and food processors.

TO STRAIN OR NOT TO STRAIN

Your baby's first feedings will need to be strained to remove any seeds, tough skins, or other hard-to-digest bits from cooked food. After cooking and pureeing the food, place a strainer over a bowl, put the food in the strainer, and with a spoon or spatula press it through the mesh. Fruits such as blueberries with skins may not strain well unless the fruit is pureed so thoroughly that the skins almost disappear. You will be surprised after peeling and chopping and pureeing that the final portion can be small. A 2-inch-diameter apple peeled, cooked, and pureed may make only 1 or 2 tablespoons of actual baby food. Cooking in batches and freezing is a time-saving and practical solution that will allow you to have food on hand at all times.

FREEZING BABY FOOD

Use clean ice cube trays to freeze batches of baby food. Fill each section with the pureed food, cover the tray with plastic wrap to keep it clean, and freeze until solid. Most foods will freeze rock hard, but some fruit purees won't freeze solid because of their natural sugar content. Once the food is frozen, remove the frozen cubes from the tray and store them in a sealed plastic bag. Keep them frozen until ready to use. Label the food so you know what it is and when you made it. Use frozen purees within a month or so.

KITCHEN EQUIPMENT BASICS

There are hundreds of utensils and pieces of equipment you could purchase for your kitchen. The following items are the tools that make cooking easy for me. I turn to these multipurpose items over and over again. Buy the best quality you can afford.

French knife: This is ideal for chopping and slicing.

Paring knife: It should have a strong, stiff blade and fit in your hand comfortably.

Set of stacking bowls: You can never have enough bowls. You'll use them for food preparation and serving.

Cutting boards: Have at least two: one for meat, chicken, and fish and one for vegetables and fruit.

Dutch oven: This is a large, heavy pot with a tight-fitting lid. It can be used to roast, stew, and boil.

10-inch skillet: Choose a pan that is heavy and has a tight-fitting lid.

Measuring cup and spoons

Set of wooden spoons: Use these for mixing and stirring.

WHAT TO COOK FIRST

There is no consensus on what foods should be fed first. Many parents choose infant cereal simply because it is well tolerated and easy to mix in small batches, often with breast milk or formula so it will taste familiar. The best foods for infants are listed alphabetically in Chapter 4, "Superior Foods."

Here is a suggested order of first foods to offer, but check with your health care provider for personalized advice.

Infant cereal
Fruit: cooked apple, ripe banana, cooked pear
Vegetables: avocado, cooked sweet potato
Meat (read about zinc and meat on page 23)

Delay wheat, citrus fruits, fish, corn, cheese, yogurt, soy, and egg yolk until six to twelve months. Delay tomatoes, egg whites, and cow's milk until twelve months. Many parents also avoid strawberries in the first year for fear they will cause allergies or skin irritations. If you have a history of food allergies in your family, talk to your doctor and read about allergy prevention on page 17. Avoid nuts, eggs, fish, cow's milk, and wheat until twelve months and possibly longer if allergies run in your family.

FIRST FOODS KIDS OFTEN LIKE BEST

The foods real mothers tell me their kids liked best, once they were old enough to have them, include apples, avocados, bananas, beans (green and dried), carrots, corn, eggs, homemade muffins, homemade soup, hummus, pears, rice cereal, spinach, and sweet potatoes. The Infant and Toddler Feeding Study found that carrots, sweet potatoes, squash, green beans, peas, and mixed garden vegetables were the most popular vegetables from four to eight months. Between nine and fourteen months green beans, mashed potatoes, french fries, mixed garden vegetables, and carrots were identified as the top five vegetables in the survey.

THREE RECIPES THAT CAN MAKE YOU
A BABY FOOD MASTER

Homemade baby food really is easy. All it takes is cooked food, a little liquid, and equipment to reduce it to a consistency that matches your child's age and development. Serve single ingredients first (refer

back to Chapter 4, "Superior Foods," for ideas on what foods to try).
The recipes that follow all make about 1 cup (sixteen 1-tablespoon
portions for freezing). Once you prepare the food, refrigerate it for
up to two days or freeze it and use within a month or so.

BASIC BABY FRUIT RECIPE

1 cup cooked or ripe fruit, skin and seeds removed if needed
1 teaspoon infant apple juice with vitamin C or lemon water
   (page 121)

Puree fruit in a food processor or food mill until it has the texture of applesauce. Refrigerate immediately or freeze.

BASIC BABY VEGETABLE RECIPE

1 cup well-cooked vegetables, skin and seeds removed if needed
4–6 tablespoons Baby Broth (page 131), formula, breast milk, or water

Puree vegetables in a food processor or food mill until they
have the texture of mayonnaise. Refrigerate or freeze.

BASIC BABY MEAT RECIPE

By the time you add these protein foods to your child's menu,
he probably will have tried a variety of fruits and vegetables.
Feel free to blend some of his favorite veggies, fruits, or cereals into this puree, especially at the beginning. Always ask
your doctor when to add protein-rich foods (including fish) to
your child's menu.

BABY'S FIRST BEEF

1 cup cooked beef
¼ cup water or Baby Broth (page 131)

Cut meat into small pieces; remove any visible fat or tough
pieces. Place in a food processor or food mill and puree with
enough liquid to achieve the desired consistency.

BABY'S FIRST CHICKEN

1 cup cooked chicken
¼ cup water or Baby Broth (page 131)

Remove any skin or fat and cut meat into chunks. Place in food processor or food mill and puree with enough liquid to achieve the desired consistency.

BABY'S FIRST FISH

½ cup cooked white boneless fish (such as haddock, cod, flounder)
2 tablespoons water or Baby Broth (page 131)

Place the fish in a food processor or food mill and puree with enough liquid to achieve the desired consistency.

WHAT'S NEXT?

After your baby has tried single-ingredient items and before you move to real table food from Chapter 6, you can use the suggestions that follow for combining ingredients to add nutrition and variety. Don't be afraid to make up your own combinations.

Any of the favorites from your child's early months can be used as she gets older. Just mix them in with lumpier ingredients so your child experiences new textures—try small cubes of cooked chicken or egg yolk.

BABY PUREES AND MASHED MIX-INS

For children six to ten months who have tasted individual foods and are ready for new combinations, try these blends. Serve them with cooked cereal, rice, or noodles, or mix in tiny pieces of chicken, egg, tofu, or beef. I give instructions for purees, but for older babies you can pulse it in the food processor or mash with a fork for a lumpy texture.

CARROT AND APRICOT

½ cup boiling water
¼ cup dried apricots
½ cup cooked carrots

Pour the boiling water over the apricots and allow to sit for 15 minutes or until fruit is soft and tender. Drain the apricots, reserving the liquid. Place the carrots in a food processor, add the apricots, and puree until smooth. Slowly add as much cooking liquid as needed to make a consistency appropriate for your child.

SWEET POTATO AND BANANA

½ cup cooked sweet potato, no skin
2-inch piece ripe banana
2 tablespoons juice, water, formula, or breast milk

Place sweet potato and banana in a food processor and puree, adding enough liquid to make a consistency appropriate for your child.

GREEN BEANS AND RICE

½ cup cooked green beans
¼ cup cooked brown or white rice
2–4 tablespoons water or Baby Broth (page 131)

Place green beans and rice in a food processor and puree, adding enough liquid to make it the desired consistency.

APPLE AND PEAR

1 apple, peeled, cored, and chopped into ½-inch cubes
1 pear, peeled, cored, and chopped into ½-inch cubes
1 tablespoon water or juice

Place the fruit and liquid in a saucepan, bring to a boil, cover, reduce heat, and simmer 3 minutes. The fruit should be soft and tender, but don't overcook or the fruit will disintegrate. Drain liquid and reserve. Place the fruit in a food processor and puree, adding liquid until it reaches the consistency appropriate for your child's age.

AVOCADO AND PEACH

1 peach
1 avocado
1 tablespoon orange juice, infant apple juice with vitamin C, or lemon
    water (below)

Peel and pit the peach, then cut the flesh into chunks. Place in a saucepan with juice, cover, and cook until tender, about 3 minutes, or microwave 1 minute. Allow to cool. Cut the avocado in half and remove the pulp. Place the peach and avocado pulp in a food processor and puree, adding liquid until the desired consistency is reached.

Lemon Water

I suggest lemon water to prevent browning of some fruits and vegetables. Mix 1 cup cold water with a teaspoon of fresh lemon juice. Cover and refrigerate and use within 7 days. Use what you need for recipes.

BANANA WITH OATMEAL

4-inch piece ripe banana
¼ cup old-fashioned oatmeal
½ cup water

Mash the banana in a bowl with the oatmeal, add water, stir, and microwave for 2 minutes, then cover and let rest for 2 minutes. (Or, on the stovetop, combine water and oats in a saucepan, bring to a boil, and simmer, covered, 3 minutes; add banana and mash.) Puree if you want a smoother consistency, adding more water, formula, or breast milk as needed.

PEAR AND POTATO

½ cup cooked potato cubes
1 ripe pear, peeled, cored, and cut into cubes
1 tablespoon juice, formula, or breast milk

Place pear and potato in food processor with liquid and puree until it reaches the appropriate consistency for your child.

FRESH FRUIT SALAD

¾ cup soft ripe fruits, skins, seeds, and membranes removed (banana, peach, and pear are good choices)
1 tablespoon fruit juice

Cut fruit into chunks. Place in a food processor, add juice, and puree, or mash with a fork for a chunkier texture.

EGG SCRAMBLES

2 egg yolks
1 tablespoon water, formula, or breast milk
2 tablespoons minced cooked green beans or carrots, or any vegetable puree you may have in the freezer
1 teaspoon oil or butter

Beat the yolks with the liquid and add vegetable. Heat a sauté pan with the oil or butter. Add egg mixture and scramble.

NEXT STEP COMBINATIONS

After ten months of age many babies have tried a variety of foods and are ready for even more textures and flavors. If this is true for your child, try the favorites that follow. However, do not feel your child is lagging behind if he still likes his single-ingredient purees. A good friend has a healthy, thriving eighteen-month-old who still likes all his veggies pureed.

MEGAN'S TOFU SPINACH PASTA SAUCE

This makes a good-size portion—enough for Mom or Dad. For the family, you can serve it over pasta with a little salt, pepper, or grated cheese added, or thin with broth for a creamier sauce if desired.

½ cup firm tofu
¼ cup cooked chopped spinach
1 teaspoon olive oil
¼ teaspoon garlic powder

Puree all ingredients until smooth. It will be very thick. Mix with well-cooked, mashed pasta.

CHICKEN AND RICE

½ cup cooked chopped chicken
⅓ cup cooked brown or white rice
¼ cup chicken broth
2 tablespoons fresh or frozen peas

Combine all ingredients in a saucepan, cover, and simmer 5 minutes, until peas are tender. Mash with a fork, chop, or pulse in a food processor to reach the consistency appropriate for your child's age.

CHICKEN AND NOODLES

Leeks give this dish a delicious taste. Make it whenever you have them on hand.

1–2 teaspoons canola oil
½ cup chopped carrot or parsnip
½ cup chopped leeks (white and light green parts) or 1 tablespoon
    minced onion or shallot
½ cup vegetable or chicken broth
¼ cup chopped chicken
½ cup cooked noodles

Heat oil and sauté vegetables about 2 minutes, until they begin to soften. Add broth, cover, and cook 5 minutes more, or until the vegetables are tender, adding a little more water if needed. Add chicken and simmer 3–4 minutes to blend flavors. Mash with a fork, chop, or pulse in the food processor to reach the consistency appropriate for your child's age. Serve with noodles.

BREAKFAST BISCUITS

MAKES 12 2-INCH BISCUITS

2 cups all-purpose flour*
1 tablespoon baking powder
¼ teaspoon salt
5 tablespoons unsalted butter, softened
½ cup milk
¼ cup maple syrup or honey

Preheat oven to 350°F. In a bowl blend dry ingredients. With clean fingers or a fork blend butter into the flour mixture until it resembles coarse meal. In a separate bowl combine milk and maple syrup. Pour over dry ingredients and stir until all the flour is moistened. Do not overmix; a few lumps are okay. Drop by spoonfuls onto a greased or parchment-lined baking sheet and bake for 18 minutes or until biscuits just start to brown.

*King Arthur unbleached flour is my favorite baking flour, but I like to mix it up by substituting rolled oats, whole cornmeal, or white whole-wheat flour for some of the white flour. Read about other grain additions on page 148.

TEETHING BISCUIT

This is a hard, dry biscuit so put it in a Baby Safe feeder to reduce the risk of choking.

2 cups flour
5 teaspoons sugar

1 egg
½–⅔ cup milk

Preheat oven to 325°F. In a bowl combine flour and sugar. In another bowl beat egg into milk. Pour egg mixture over flour and mix well. Press into 8 × 8″ pan. Bake 45 minutes. Cut into squares before they cool.

OVERNIGHT BREAKFAST PORRIDGE

Serve this after the first birthday because of the cow's milk.

¼ cup rolled oats
¼ cup white rice
2 tablespoons raisins, chopped
¾ cup water
¾ cup whole milk

Combine oats, rice, raisins, and water. Let soak 3 hours or overnight in the refrigerator. In a small saucepan heat the grain mixture, add the milk, and simmer until the liquid is absorbed and the rice and oats are tender, about 10–20 minutes. Allow to cool a bit. Serve as is or process in a food processor until the raisins are in tiny pieces.

LENTIL STEW

1 teaspoon canola oil or olive oil
¼ cup grated parsnips
¼ cup grated carrots
2 cups vegetable broth
1 cup red or green lentils, picked over and rinsed
1 small potato, peeled and diced or grated (about ½ cup)
1 teaspoon lemon juice

Heat oil and sauté parsnips and carrots. Add ¼ cup broth and cook until tender, about 5 minutes. Add remaining broth, lentils, and potato and cook on low heat for 30 minutes, or until potato and lentils are tender. Add lemon juice. Mash with a fork, chop, or pulse in the food processor to reach the consistency appropriate for your child's age.

VEGETABLE PUDDING

The addition of egg makes this a complete meal. If using whole eggs, serve only after your child's first birthday because of the egg white.

1 teaspoon butter
1 teaspoon flour
⅓ cup milk
½ cup pureed vegetables, such as carrots, beets, green beans, and/or spinach
1 egg, beaten, or 2 egg yolks

Preheat the oven to 350°F. Lightly grease two custard cups. In a small saucepan melt the butter, add the flour, and cook 2 minutes. Add milk and cook, stirring, until the mixture is smooth. Remove from heat. Stir in the vegetable puree, then mix in the egg. Pour into custard cups and bake 20 minutes. Mash with a fork, chop, or pulse in the food processor to reach the consistency appropriate for your child's age.

YOGURT WITH PRUNE SAUCE

2 prunes, pitted and chopped
¼ cup boiling water
½ cup plain whole-milk yogurt

In a small bowl combine prunes with boiling water. Allow to steep for 15 minutes or until prunes are plump and rehydrated. Drain, reserving liquid. Puree the prunes with enough reserved liquid to make a smooth sauce. Pour the sauce over the yogurt and serve.

TWELVE TO EIGHTEEN MONTHS

These recipes use seasonings including bay leaf, oregano, cumin, and parsley, but still no salt.

BABY REFRIED BEANS

1 tablespoon canola oil
1 tablespoon minced onion
One 15½ -ounce can no-salt-added kidney or black beans, drained and
   rinsed, or 1½ cups home-cooked beans
¼ cup water

In a small saucepan heat the oil and cook onion until tender, about 4 minutes. Add beans and water, mashing the beans with the back of a fork. Cook for 5 minutes, until heated through and some of the water has evaporated. The beans will thicken as they cool. Serve with rice or cooked vegetables.

Rinsing canned beans can remove salt, but it does not remove protein.

LISA'S VEGGIE AND CHICKPEA STEW

This makes enough for Mom and Dad's lunch or dinner, too. Just season the adults' with a little pepper or grated cheese.

1 tablespoon olive oil
1 medium onion, chopped
2 carrots, peeled and diced (about 1 cup)
1 celery stalk, diced (about ½ cup)
2 garlic cloves, minced
½ teaspoon rosemary
¼ teaspoon thyme
1 bay leaf
2 cups water
2 tablespoons tomato paste

Two 15½-ounce cans chickpeas, drained and rinsed, or 1½ cup home-cooked
2 cups broccoli/cauliflower mix

Heat oil in a large saucepan. Add onion and cook until soft, 4–5 minutes. Add carrot, celery, garlic, rosemary, thyme, and bay leaf and cook 5 minutes more. Stir in water, tomato paste, and chickpeas. Cook 30 minutes. Discard bay leaf. Remove 1 cup of mixture from pot and puree. Return puree to stew. Reduce heat, stir in broccoli and cauliflower, and cook 7 minutes, until the vegetables mash easily. Add ½ to 1 cup water if it looks dry. Mash with a fork, chop, or pulse in a food processor to reach the consistency appropriate for your child's age.

LISA'S BEAN, CORN, AND ZUCCHINI STEW

Enough for the whole family. Serve with good bread.

1 tablespoon olive oil
½ cup brown rice
1 medium onion, diced
1 garlic clove, minced
Two 14½-ounce cans vegetable or chicken broth or 3 cups homemade broth (see Baby Broth, page 131)
1 medium zucchini, diced (about 2 cups)
2 cups frozen corn kernels
One 15½-ounce can pinto or light red kidney beans, drained and rinsed
½ teaspoon oregano
¼ teaspoon cumin
⅛ teaspoon finely ground pepper (optional)

In an 8-cup saucepan heat oil. Add rice, onion, and garlic and cook 2–3 minutes, until onion is tender. Add remaining ingredients. Bring to a boil, then reduce heat, cover, and simmer 45 minutes, until rice is tender. Add more liquid if too thick. Mash with a fork, chop, or pulse in the food processor to reach the consistency appropriate for your child's age.

CHICKEN BARLEY STEW

Dark meat makes the most flavorful stews and casseroles.

Two boneless, skinless chicken thighs, chopped
1 cup water or broth
½ cup brown rice or barley
½ cup chopped carrots
½ cup chopped green beans

Combine all ingredients in a 4-cup saucepan. Bring to a boil, stir, reduce heat, and cover. Simmer 45 minutes, until the rice or barley is very tender. Add more water or broth if it looks dry. Mash with a fork, chop, or pulse in the food processor to reach the consistency appropriate for your child's age. Or remove chicken, puree the chicken, and stir back into the stew.

IMAGINATION SOUP

1 cup baby broth (chicken, vegetable, or beef) (see page 131)
½ cup chopped carrot, parsnip, turnip, or potato
½ cup chopped green beans, peas, broccoli, or asparagus tips
¼ cup chopped canned tomato
¼ cup frozen or fresh corn kernels
¼ cup chopped onion or leeks
½ cup chickpeas or kidney beans (optional)
1 bay leaf

In a 4-cup saucepan combine all ingredients. Bring to a boil, reduce heat, cover, and simmer 30 minutes, until the vegetables are all very tender. Remove bay leaf before serving.

Imagination Soup with Beef or Chicken: Follow the above recipe and add ½ cup chopped cooked beef (leftover pot roast is a delicious addition) or chicken to the broth and vegetables.

BABY'S FIRST BEEF STEW

½ cup water or vegetable broth
½ cup cubed cooked beef
¼ cup cubed peeled potato
2 tablespoons frozen peas
2 tablespoons chopped carrots
1 tablespoon finely chopped celery

Heat 1 cup water or broth in a saucepan. Add beef and vegetables. Simmer 20 minutes, adding more liquid as needed. All the vegetables should be very soft, and the beef should be very tender. Mash with a fork, chop, or pulse in the food processor to reach the consistency appropriate for your child's age.

CREAMED CHICKEN

1 tablespoon butter
1 tablespoon flour
½–¾ cup whole milk
¼ cup chopped cooked chicken

Melt butter in a small saucepan, stir in flour, and cook 2 minutes until it looks like wet paste. Slowly add ½ cup milk, stirring constantly until smooth. Mix in chicken and add remaining ¼ cup milk to make it creamier (if desired).

Serve creamed chicken over rice or pasta. Fold in cooked vegetable if desired.

TWICE BAKED CREAMED FISH

½ cup yellow beans or cooked carrots
½ cup cooked whitefish, chopped
½ cup mashed potato

Preheat oven to 350°F. In a small bowl puree the beans or carrots. Fold in the whitefish and mashed potato. Put the mixture into a lightly oiled ramekin or a ½-cup custard cup and bake for 20 minutes. Cool before serving.

BABY BROTH—CHICKEN, VEGETABLE, AND BEEF

Making homemade broth is very easy, and it is far, far superior to canned products, which almost always have an excessive amount of sodium. Keep broth in the freezer in individual and 1 cup portions, and you will be able to make baby stews and soups that are perfect in nutrition and texture for your child. Try the recipe for Imagination Soup on page 129 using your child's favorite ingredients. If you must used canned broth, read about Broth in "Superior Foods" on page 69.

CHICKEN BROTH

1½ pounds chicken wings (about 6 wings)
1 onion, chopped
2 celery stalks with leaves cut into 3-inch pieces
1 bay leaf
10 sprigs fresh parsley

Bring 5 cups cold water to a boil. Add chicken wings, onion, celery, bay leaf, and parsley. Return to a boil and skim any foam that rises to the top. Stir, cover, and simmer for 30–60 minutes.

Remove chicken wings. Allow broth to cool at room temperature, strain, then refrigerate until cold and remove congealed fat from the surface. Refrigerate for 2 days, or pour into 1-tablespoon portions in ice cube trays or 1–4 cup containers.

Remove meat from the chicken wings, and use in other recipes. It can be kept refrigerated for up to 2 days or frozen for use at a later time.

FRESH VEGETABLE BROTH

3 cloves garlic, peeled and smashed with the blade of a knife
2 celery ribs, chopped into chunks (include the leaves)
8 ounces fresh mushrooms, whole or sliced
1 cup peeled and chopped carrots
2 cups leeks, cut into chunks (optional but delicious)
2 large potatoes, cubed
10 sprigs fresh flat leaf parsley
2 tablespoons fresh rosemary, dill, or thyme
1 bay leaf
10 black peppercorns
1 large onion, peeled and quartered
8–10 cups cold water
1 teaspoon dry thyme, ground
¼ teaspoon ground clove

Rinse all vegetables and fresh herbs. Fill a pot with the water and add all ingredients except the last two (thyme and clove). Bring to a boil, reduce heat to low, and simmer covered for 1 hour.

Remove cover, stir in remaining two ingredients, and simmer uncovered another 30 minutes. Line a colander with cheesecloth and strain broth. Remove the cooked carrots and potatoes and serve as part of another meal. Allow the broth to cool, then refrigerate or freeze.

SECOND HARVEST STOCK

This recipe uses a ratio of 1 cup water to 1 cup leftover vegetable trimmings to make an economical and delicious stock.

2 cups chopped green leek tops
2 cups parsley stems
2 cups green vegetable trimmings (any combination of broccoli stalks, empty pea pods, wilted greens from escarole, endive, spinach, or celery leaves)
6 cups cold water

1 bay leaf
2 carrots, chopped
½ teaspoon salt
1 tablespoon fresh thyme or oregano

In a large pot combine all ingredients except the thyme or oregano. Bring to a boil, stir, and simmer uncovered for 30 minutes. Stir in fresh herbs, and simmer 5–10 minutes more. Pour through a strainer. Cool and keep refrigerated until ready to use or freeze in 1-cup portions.

BEEF BROTH

3 pounds beef bones (ask your butcher to crack the bones to enhance the flavor)
2 quarts cold water
1 bay leaf
1 teaspoon ground thyme
¼ cup flat parsley, chopped
1 large carrot, chopped
2 stalks celery, chopped, including leaves
1 large onion, chopped
1 teaspoon salt

Cook the bones in a 350°F oven for about 1 hour or until browned. Place bones in a large stockpot with the drippings and cover with water. Bring to a boil and simmer for 30 minutes uncovered. Remove foam as it rises to the surface.

Add remaining ingredients, and cook uncovered for 3–5 hours or until broth has reduced to about 6 cups. Allow to cool, then remove bones and strain the stock. Refrigerate or freeze in an ice cube tray or as 1-cup or 4-cup portions.

USING A PRESSURE COOKER

Chicken, Fresh Vegetable, Second Harvest, and Beef broths can all be prepared using a pressure cooker. Put all ingredients in the pressure cooker. Follow the manufacturer's guidelines regarding amount of water and do not exceed the recommended limit. Cook on high pressure for 20 minutes. When cool enough to remove top, stir in ground herbs. Strain through cheesecloth as directed above.

A Guide to Food Consistency by Age

Below are very general guidelines for matching the right food consistency with your child's age. Check with your health care provider for his or her recommendations.

Age	Food Form
Birth–4 months	liquid
4–6 months	strained
6–8 months	strained to mashed
8–10 months	mashed to minced
10–12 months	minced to chopped
12–36 months	chopped table food

Are You Worried About Your Child's Sweet Tooth?

Children like the taste of sweet food; this is normal. In the first twelve to fifteen months you can satisfy your child's desire for sweet tastes with fruit—cooked, raw, or in baked food. After eighteen months if you are serving dessert or sweet food, keep the portions small and serve as part of a meal or a snack. If you don't allow sweets to crowd out other nutritious foods, you won't have a problem.

You Should Worry About Your Child's Salt Tooth!

Your child is born with a sweet tooth, but he will learn to have a salt tooth. Many packaged foods, including cereals and crackers, are excessively high in salt. Learning to like salty foods early on increases the desire for salt later on, and most of the time foods high in salt are inferior foods that replace foods that promote health. Read labels and save salty foods like french fries and potato chips for special occasions. Read more about salt and inferior foods on page 57.

SIX

The Family Table

After your baby's first birthday, you can transition her to table food quite nicely. Since you have to cook for yourself and other family members, why not make something that works for everyone? If you are preparing wholesome meals that include a variety of foods and your recipes minimize salt, your meals can be chopped, mashed, or pureed for your growing baby.

"I keep feeding her the same thing. I don't want to give her something that is too spicy, so I make something for me and my husband and give her macaroni and cheese." Whether it's macaroni and cheese, chicken tenders, cereal, pizza, or peanut butter and jelly sandwiches, this is one of the most common remarks I hear from parents about feeding young children. If you don't serve your child the food you eat, she will not be learning to eat well. Don't hold back—prepare good food, then share it. Keep in mind that children in other countries have taste preferences for very different foods, including fermented cabbage, chile peppers, and tofu, simply because those are the foods their family eats and the ones they were fed as children. To help your child be more adventurous, serve her what you eat, and include three or more items at every meal. Always provide at least one food you know she will like, and include a fruit, a vegetable, or both.

This chapter includes more than fifty of my favorite everyday family recipes, all appropriate for a young child if they are pureed, mashed, or chopped to a consistency that meets her eating ability. The main dish recipes for beef, poultry, or fish will probably all look familiar to you, but they are designed for the family feeding young children, so they are prepared without any unnecessary salt; instead, herbs and vegetables are used for flavoring. Main-dish recipes yield four adult-size portions. Baked goods are easy to make, and I hope they will encourage you to cook with whole grains such as whole-wheat flour or oats, the foods that really do extend life and add a dimension of flavor not available in store-bought goods. Finally, the everyday desserts included in this book are fruit-based or made with whole grains and other simple, natural ingredients.

These recipes are also easy—they use common ingredients and include as few steps as possible. When you want to prepare something more elaborate, go to your favorite cookbook and adjust the recipes to make them appropriate for young children—eliminate or reduce salt, cook all meats thoroughly, and don't use very hot spices. If you are stuck in a rut, subscribe to one of the many food magazines—I particularly like *Gourmet* and *Fine Cooking*. My favorite Web pages include www.foodnetwork.com and www.epicurious.com.

My recipes rarely add salt, and when it is used, amounts are very small. If you have family members who want more salt, have them add it at the table—don't add it to the recipe. To plan meals, use the foods suggested in Chapter 4, "Superior Foods," as side dishes. See the Vegetable Cooking Primer on page 171 for a review of how to steam, bake, or roast vegetables.

EVERYDAY APPETIZERS

Every family should be sharing family meals as often as possible. However, there is a limit to how long infants or toddlers can be expected to sit at a table, or how peaceful a meal will be when they are at the table! The recipes that follow can be used as appetizers for adults; served with a glass of milk, fruit, and a slice of bread, they can become a full dinner for children. You can eat these with your child, and once he goes to bed, you can have a quiet dinner with your partner or friends. Because these appetizers are all vegetable-based, they won't add up to too many calories when paired with an entree.

HUMMUS

A delicious dip or sandwich spread. Serve it only to a child who has already eaten seeds or nuts with no reaction. *For young children:* This is a good protein food. Serve with vegetables and/or a little rice or noodles for a complete meal. Don't serve thin crisp crackers to very young children, however, as pieces can break off and become a choking hazard.

One 15½-ounce can chickpeas, drained and rinsed, or 1½ cups well-cooked chickpeas
½ cup tahini (sesame seed paste, available in most supermarkets) or peanut butter
1 teaspoon minced garlic
1 tablespoon cumin
Juice of 1 lemon
Olive oil
Pinch of salt

Combine beans, tahini or peanut butter, garlic, cumin, and lemon juice in a processor. Puree, adding enough olive oil to make a smooth paste. Add a little water if you want it thinner. Season with salt if desired. Serve with thin-sliced bread, pita, or crackers.

EGGPLANT CAVIAR

Cooked eggplant has a funny color but a delicate flavor and a creamy, soft texture. *For young children:* This recipe contains both yogurt and vegetables, so just add bread or noodles and a glass of milk for a well-balanced meal. *For Mom and Dad:* Season with salt and pepper to taste and eat as a dip.

1 large eggplant (1½ pounds)
Olive oil
1 teaspoon chopped garlic
Juice of half a lemon
4 tablespoons whole-milk yogurt or cottage cheese
1 large tomato, peeled and chopped (optional)

Heat the oven to 400°F. Cut the eggplant in half and brush with olive oil. Place cut side down in a baking dish and cook 40 minutes or until very soft. Let cool. With a spoon scoop out the cooked pulp. Place half of the pulp in a food processor with the garlic and lemon juice and puree until smooth. Add the remaining eggplant and pulse until the mixture is smooth but still a little chunky. Place in a bowl and stir in yogurt and tomato. Serve with pita or other bread.

Note: This does not freeze well.

GUACAMOLE

Many recipes for guacamole are made with chile peppers. Here mild chili powder is substituted. *For young children:* Serve this with cooked beans and rice or a soft tortilla and a slice of fruit. *For Mom and Dad:* Serve with tortillas and salsa of your choice.

2 ripe avocados
Juice of 1 lemon
1 scallion, finely minced
1 tablespoon fresh minced cilantro (optional)
⅛ teaspoon mild chili powder
1 cup chopped tomato (optional)
1 small cucumber, peeled and chopped (optional)

Scoop out avocado, and mash with lemon juice. Stir in remaining ingredients. Refrigerate, covered tightly with plastic wrap, or serve immediately.

FRUIT AND VEGETABLES FOR DIPPING

Most of us turn to crackers or chips when serving dips, but these do nothing to improve your health, and they don't set a good example for your child. Consider serving dips with fruits or vegetables most of the time, and save the chips and crackers for parties and special occasions. If you do not like raw vegetables, bring 2 quarts of water to a boil, add any of the vegetables listed below, and cook for 3 minutes. Drain and run under cold water to stop the cooking. You want the vegetables tender but not so cooked they fall apart.

Any of the following are dipping possibilities:

Asparagus
Carrot sticks
Sugar snap peas or snow peas
Broccoli florets
Cauliflower florets
Bell peppers of all colors

Fresh ripe fruit can also be used for dips. Consider these:

Melon slices
Orange wedges
Sliced grapes
Blueberries
Banana
Apple slices dipped in lemon water (page 121)

YOGURT AVOCADO DIP

1 small ripe avocado
2 tablespoons lemon juice
½ cup plain yogurt (low-fat or whole-milk)

Peel and mash the avocado with the lemon juice. Stir in the yogurt and blend until very smooth. Add more yogurt if you want it thinner.

VERY BERRY DIP

Serve with sliced fruit.

1 cup frozen raspberries or strawberries
1 cup vanilla whole-milk yogurt

Puree the berries in a food processor and strain to remove seeds. Mix with yogurt. Refrigerate until ready to serve.

PEANUT BUTTER DIP

For young children: Serve as a dip with vegetables or on top of cooked noodles. *For Mom and Dad:* Use as a dip with blanched broccoli, asparagus tips, or sugar snap peas.

½ cup smooth peanut butter
1 teaspoon sesame oil
1 teaspoon canola oil
3 tablespoons orange juice
1 teaspoon soy sauce (for Mom and Dad)

Combine all ingredients except soy sauce. Remove half the recipe for your baby and add soy sauce to the rest for the adults. Whisk until smooth. Refrigerate until ready to serve.

YOGURT CHEESE DIP

1 quart plain whole-milk yogurt

Layer a colander with three thicknesses of cheesecloth and place it over a bowl. Fill the colander with the yogurt, place a weighted bowl or plate on top of the yogurt, and refrigerate overnight. The water will drip out and you will be left with a yummy cream-cheese-like concoction that you can mix with herbs, spices, and minced vegetables and spread on crackers. Or turn it into a dessert by blending it with a little cinnamon, a dash of vanilla, a teaspoon of brown sugar, and some cooked or ripe chopped fruit.

What Is Wrong with Cheese and Crackers?

Cheese and crackers is an American snack staple, but don't serve it every day. Two ounces of sliced cheese and eight crackers will provide about 300 calories, 16 grams of saturated fat (20 grams is a day's amount for adults), and more than half a day's supply of sodium. If Mom and Dad start the dinner hour with a high-fat, high-calorie appetizer like this, they will be gaining weight and raising their cholesterol. Young children love cheese, but it is a high-fat way to get calcium, and it can replace the foods that improve health, such as fruit and vegetables. Serve cheese in small amounts as part of meals, and when it is served as a snack, combine it with sliced fruit.

ONE-BOWL BAKING

I love to cook. Give me a cool, stormy day with hours of unscheduled time and I am likely to spend it baking an elaborate cake. But in the morning, when the family has a busy schedule that starts at 6:30 A.M., I turn to my one-bowl favorites. These are baked goods that lose nothing by being prepared quickly and efficiently, and they are a great alternative to store-bought muffins or white-flour pancake and baking mixes. The trick to one-bowl baking is not to overmix the batter—it should be a little lumpy, not smooth like a cake batter. Also, measure the dry ingredients first and mix well so the baking powder or baking soda is evenly distributed in the flour.

Muffins

A perfect snack and a great way to add fruit and vegetables to your child's diet. Homemade muffins are far superior to the ones made with high-fructose corn syrup, fake fruit, and white flour. Make and freeze a batch of these so you always have some on hand.

SIMPLE MUFFINS

MAKES 6 MUFFINS

1 cup all-purpose flour
2 teaspoons baking powder
¼ teaspoon salt
2 tablespoons sugar
½ cup milk
1 egg
2 tablespoons canola oil or melted butter

Preheat oven to 375°F. Grease a muffin pan, or use paper liners. Combine flour, baking powder, salt, and sugar in a medium-size bowl. Mix well. Form a well in the center of the flour mixture and add the milk, egg, and oil. Stir by hand just until the wet and dry ingredients are blended. Fill each muffin cup about two-thirds full. Bake 15–20 minutes, until the tops are golden brown.

Oatmeal Muffins: Substitute ½ cup quick-cooking oatmeal for half the flour. This makes a very textured muffin. For a smooth muffin, grind ½ cup rolled oats in a food processor, measure, and add enough all-purpose flour to make 1 cup.

ZUCCHINI MUFFINS

1 cup all-purpose flour
2 teaspoons baking powder
¼ teaspoon salt
2 tablespoons sugar
½ teaspoon cinnamon
¼ teaspoon ground cloves
¼ teaspoon freshly grated nutmeg
½ cup milk
1 egg
½ cup finely grated zucchini
2 tablespoons canola oil

Preheat oven to 375°F. Grease a muffin pan or use paper liners. Mix flour, baking powder, salt, sugar, cinnamon, cloves, and nutmeg. Form a well in the center of the flour mixture and add the milk, egg, zucchini, and oil. Stir by hand just until the wet and dry ingredients are blended. Fill each muffin cup about two-thirds full. Bake 15–20 minutes, until the tops are golden brown.

BANANA MUFFINS

1 cup all-purpose flour
2 teaspoons baking powder
¼ teaspoon salt
2–4 tablespoons sugar (use the larger portion of sugar for a sweeter muffin)
½ teaspoon cinnamon
½ cup milk
1 egg
1 small banana, mashed, about ½ cup
2 tablespoons canola oil

Preheat oven to 425°F. Grease a muffin pan or use paper liners. Mix flour, baking powder, salt, sugar, and cinnamon. Form a well in the center of the flour mixture and add milk, egg, banana, and oil.

Stir by hand just until the wet and dry ingredients are blended. Fill each muffin cup about two-thirds full. Bake 15–20 minutes, until the tops are golden brown.

BLUEBERRY MUFFINS

MAKES 6 MUFFINS

1 cup all-purpose flour
2 teaspoons baking powder
¼ teaspoon salt
2 tablespoons sugar
½ teaspoon cinnamon

½ cup milk
1 egg
2 tablespoons canola oil
½ cup fresh or frozen blueberries

Preheat oven to 425°F. Grease a muffin pan or use paper liners. Mix flour, baking powder, salt, sugar, and cinnamon. Make a well in the flour mixture and add the milk, egg, and oil. Stir just until the wet and dry ingredients are blended.

Fold blueberries gently into the batter. Fill each muffin cup about two-thirds full. Bake 15–20 minutes, until the tops are golden brown.

Variation: To make Peach Muffins, substitute ½ cup chopped peeled peaches for the blueberries.

WHOLE-GRAIN MUFFINS

Follow the recipe for any of the muffins above, substituting ½ cup whole-wheat flour for ½ cup of the all-purpose flour, or 1 cup whole-wheat pastry flour for all the all-purpose flour. Read about flour substitutions on page 148.

CARROT PINEAPPLE MUFFINS

This makes a moist muffin your whole family will enjoy. Even those who do not like pineapple will like this recipe as the carrots and pineapple blend into the oats to make a delicious warm treat.

⅔ cup all-purpose flour
½ cup rolled oats
¾ teaspoon baking powder
½ teaspoon baking soda
½ teaspoon cinnamon
⅛ teaspoon ground cloves
½ cup sugar
½ cup oil

2 eggs, lightly beaten
⅔ cup grated carrot
One 8½ ounce can crushed pineapple, drained

Preheat oven to 350°F. In a large bowl combine first six ingredients. Add sugar, oil, eggs, carrot, and pineapple, and mix until blended. Do not overmix.

Spoon batter into a 12-cup muffin pan with paper liners. Bake 18 to 22 minutes until lightly browned on top. Remove muffins from pan and let cool 10 minutes on a wire rack before serving.

Buttermilk or Sour Milk Muffins and Pancakes

For a change of flavor and texture in any of the muffin or pancake recipes, try using buttermilk or sour milk in place of regular milk. To make sour milk, add 1 teaspoon white vinegar to ½ cup milk and let it sit for 3 minutes. It will curdle slightly and offers a delicious, subtle change in flavor.

CORN MUFFINS

½ cup all-purpose flour
½ cup cornmeal
2 teaspoons baking powder
½ teaspoon salt
2 tablespoons sugar
½ cup milk
1 egg
2 tablespoons melted butter

Preheat oven to 425°F. Grease a muffin pan or use paper liners. Combine flour, cornmeal, baking powder, salt, and sugar. Form a well in the center of the flour mixture and add milk, egg, and butter. Stir by hand just until the wet and dry ingredients are blended. Fill each muffin cup about two-thirds full. Bake 15–20 minutes, until the tops are golden brown.

Pancakes

Like muffins, pancakes can be a great way to eat whole grains and fruit. This recipe makes about twelve 4-inch pancakes. Cook up a batch and use leftovers for snacks, or freeze for a quick breakfast on another day. To freeze pancakes, put them in a single layer on a baking sheet in the freezer. Once frozen, transfer to a plastic bag and keep frozen until ready to reheat in the microwave or oven.

BASIC PANCAKES

2 cups all-purpose flour
1 teaspoon baking powder
¼ teaspoon salt
1 tablespoon sugar
2 eggs
1½ cups milk, warmed slightly
2 tablespoons melted butter or canola oil

Mix flour, baking powder, salt, and sugar. Add the eggs, milk, and butter to the dry ingredients and stir just until moistened. Heat an electric griddle or large skillet. Grease if not using a nonstick pan. Pour ¼ cup batter onto the hot griddle. Cook 2–4 minutes a side, until bubbles appear on the top. Flip and cook another 1–3 minutes. Serve warm.

Berry Pancakes: Use 1 cup frozen or fresh blueberries or strawberries (chop the strawberries into ½-inch pieces). Sprinkle the berries over the batter as soon as it is poured onto the griddle.

Cornmeal Pancakes: Substitute 1 cup whole cornmeal for 1 cup flour and proceed as directed. Try this recipe combined with blueberries.

Banana Pancakes: Mix 1 cup mashed ripe banana (about two small bananas) into the wet ingredients before proceeding.

Flour Substitutions

Today's cook has a variety of flours to choose from, and it can be fun and delicious to experiment with them. All-purpose flour produces superior baked goods because of its protein content and subtle flavor. I often replace some of the all-purpose flour called for in recipes with whole-grain flour. Flour made from whole grains makes a denser product and does not rise as much but has more nutrients. If you like a more traditional texture, try using whole-wheat pastry flour, which is more finely milled and seems to bake more like white flour. I also like King Arthur white whole-wheat flour (see page 124). When cooking with whole grains, start by replacing only one-quarter to one-half of the flour called for with whole-grain flour.

You can even make your own whole-grain flour with ingredients you have at home. Raw oats, brown rice, and barley can all be ground into flour using a coffee mill or electric grinder. I have used my mini-food processor to make flour, too, but it takes a little longer and the final result is not as fine as when I use my coffee grinder. A half cup of any of these grains will yield about ½ cup of flour that can replace some of the flour in any of the recipes listed here.

If you want to learn more about whole-grain cooking, I highly recommend *King Arthur Flour Whole Grain Baking*. Every recipe I have tried in that book has been perfect. For additional information on whole-grain cooking and nutrition, contact the Whole Grains Council, www.wholegrainscouncil.org.

Gluten-Free Baking and Cooking

Some families need a gluten-free diet because they have family members with sensitivity to a naturally occurring protein called gluten. Gluten is found in wheat, rye, and barley. Such a restriction calls for new ways of cooking, as wheat is used not only in baking but also to make gravies and sauces. Read more about a gluten-free diet on page 218.

Grains Containing Gluten

Wheat (including spelt, kamut, semolina, triticale)
Rye
Barley

Gluten-Free Grains

Rice
Amaranth
Buckwheat
Corn
Millet
Quinoa
Sorghum
Teff (an Ethiopian grain)
*Oats**

Sources of Gluten-Free Starches That Can Be Used as Flour Alternatives

Cereal grains: amaranth, buckwheat, corn, millet, montina (Indian rice grass), quinoa, rice, sorghum, teff, rice
Tubers: arrowroot, jicama, taro, potato, tapioca (cassava, manioc, yucca)
Legumes: chickpeas, lentils, kidney beans, navy beans, pea beans, peanuts, soybeans
Nuts: almonds, walnuts, chestnuts, hazelnuts, cashews
Seeds: sunflower, flax, pumpkin

*Oats are often processed in the same plants that handle wheat, potentially causing cross-contamination. If you're avoiding gluten, check the label for a statement that the oats are gluten-free.

PANCAKE TOPPING

Instead of smothering pancakes with syrup and butter, try this fruit topping, or use Very Berry Dip on page 141 as a topping. These are good for the whole family.

2 apples, peeled, cored, and chopped (about 1 cup), or 1 cup frozen or
  fresh blueberries
1 tablespoon pure maple syrup
1 tablespoon water or juice
¼ teaspoon cinnamon

Combine all ingredients in a small saucepan. Cover and cook for 10 minutes, or until berries burst or apples are very soft.

MY MOTHER'S BREAD

My mother, Elizabeth Jane Hall Behan, was a terrific cook and an exceptional bread baker. This is her family recipe, and I have used it countless times to feed hungry kids. These days I use a blend of white and whole-wheat flour.

3 cups warm water
3 tablespoons yeast
¼ cup honey
9–10 cups all-purpose flour, or 4 cups whole-wheat and 5–6 cups all-
  purpose white
5 teaspoons salt
5 tablespoons canola oil

Combine water, yeast, and honey and stir until yeast dissolves. Let sit in a warm spot to proof, until a soft spongy layer forms on the surface. This takes about 5–10 minutes. Add half the flour and all the salt. Beat hard with a spoon until the batter is smooth. Add the remaining flour and blend well. Pour oil over dough and knead in the bowl for 2–3 minutes, until the dough has absorbed most of the oil. Cover bowl and let rise in a warm place until doubled, about 45 minutes. Punch down and turn out onto a lightly floured board. Knead slightly.

Shape into two loaves and put into greased bread pans. Cover and let rise until doubled, about 30 minutes. Bake in a pre-heated 400°F oven for 30 minutes. When done, it should be lightly browned and sound hollow when tapped. Cool 5 minutes, then remove from pan and set on cooling rack until ready to slice.

EVERYDAY LUNCH

QUESADILLA WITH VEGETABLES

This makes a warm, quick sandwich. *For young children:* Cut into small wedges, and always choose vegetables that will be easy to chew when well cooked.

½ cup grated Monterey Jack or cheddar cheese
½ cup cooked chopped peppers, carrot, broccoli, or other vegetable
½ cup chopped cooked chicken or Baby Refried Beans (page 127)
4 flour tortillas

Combine the cheese, vegetables, and chicken or beans in a bowl. Sprinkle one-fourth of the mixture on half of each tortilla. Fold tortillas in half.

Lightly oil a frying pan. Cook tortillas one at a time over high heat, about 1 one minute a side, until warm and cheese has melted. Cut into wedges. Serve plain or with chopped tomato or homemade salsa.

CALZONE

Make a batch of these and keep them in the freezer. Thaw and bake, and you will have a well-fed and happy family in no time at all. *For young children:* Cut calzone into bite-size pieces. Choose a mild, well-liked cheese, and experiment with different vegetables.

1 pound frozen bread dough or prepared pizza dough, thawed
½ cup chopped cooked chicken or 4 ounces sliced chicken

*½–1 cup cooked vegetables, your choice (I like shredded carrot,
  zucchini that's been squeezed to get rid of excess water, or cooked
  chopped peppers)*
½ cup shredded cheese

On a floured surface, roll dough into an 8-by-14-inch rectangle. If it is hard to roll, let it rest 5 minutes, pick it up by one edge, and shake it as if it were a blanket on the beach, then try rolling it again. In a small bowl combine the chicken, vegetable, and cheese. Spread the mixture over three-quarters of the rolled-out dough, leaving at least 2 inches of untouched dough along one of the 14-inch edges. Starting at the vegetable/chicken-covered long edge, roll up and press to seal. Place on a lightly oiled or nonstick baking pan. Form into a circle and cut ten evenly spaced slashes in the dough. This makes it easier to cut when cooked.

Cover and let the dough rise in a warm spot for 15 minutes. Meanwhile, preheat the oven to 350°F. Bake 25 minutes or until lightly browned.

Sandwich Ideas

I love sandwiches because they are the original fast food. Make them with a whole-grain bread and a lean filling and serve with chopped vegetables inside or on the side, and you have a good meal. Wrap them in foil or plastic and they can travel with you to a friend's house or play date. Cut into appropriate-size pieces for your child.

Here are some of my favorite fillings:

Peanut butter
Chicken
Lean meats, chopped
*Canned light tuna mixed with a small amount of mayonnaise (try it
  with yogurt instead of mayonnaise, or a combination)*
Canned salmon (prepared like tuna)
Chopped egg with a little mayonnaise and yogurt

EVERYDAY SOUP

Soup is an easy and delicious way to combine healthful ingredients such as whole grains, vegetables, and earth-friendly protein choices. Assemble all the ingredients and while the soup simmers you can take care of the baby, or if you're really lucky, you can put your feet up and read.

VEGETABLE BARLEY SOUP

1 tablespoon canola oil
1 pound sliced mushrooms
4 cups vegetable or chicken broth (see pages 131–132)
½ cup pearl barley
2 cups grated carrot
1 large bay leaf

In a 2-quart pot, heat the oil and sauté the mushrooms until soft, about 1 minute. Add ¼ cup broth and cook another 3 minutes. Add all remaining ingredients, cover, and simmer 45–60 minutes, until the barley is soft. Remove bay leaf.

CHICKEN (OR TURKEY) AND RICE SOUP

Nothing beats this soup for busy moms and hungry kids. It takes 1 hour to cook, but all you really do is put everything in a pot and let the stovetop do the work. Adults can season their portion with salt and pepper if desired.

1 quart chicken broth (see page 131)
½ cup brown rice
2 large carrots, peeled and chopped
1 celery stalk, chopped very fine
¼ cup chopped flat parsley (optional)
2 cups chopped cooked chicken or turkey

Combine the broth, rice, and vegetables in a large pot. Simmer for 45 minutes. Add the chicken and cook 15 minutes more, until the rice and vegetables are very soft.

CHICKPEA, LENTIL, AND RICE SOUP

Lentils cook in the same amount of time as rice, but dried chickpeas take much longer, so I use the canned version.

1 tablespoon olive oil
1 onion, chopped
1 clove garlic, minced
¼ teaspoon oregano
One 15-ounce can no-salt-added chickpeas
½ cup lentils, picked over and rinsed
½ cup brown rice
1 tablespoon tomato paste
One 14-ounce can diced tomatoes
4 cups baby broth (see page 131)

In a large pot heat the oil and cook onion about 4–5 minutes, until soft. Add garlic and cook 1 minute more. Stir in all remaining ingredients. Bring to a boil, then reduce heat and simmer, covered, for 45–50 minutes, until the rice and lentils are very tender.

LEEK SOUP

Leeks must be very well washed to remove any grit or dirt that may have found its way between the vegetable's layers.

2 tablespoons butter
2 cups chopped leeks (white and green parts from 3 leeks)
1 onion, chopped
2 large potatoes, peeled and chopped (about 1 cup)
1 cup water
½ cup chicken or vegetable broth (see pages 131–132)
2 cups whole milk

In a large pot melt the butter, add the leeks and onion, and cook 10 minutes, covered, over low heat. Add potatoes and water and cook 30 minutes more, until the potatoes are tender. Puree the mixture in batches in a blender or food processor. Return the mixture to the pot. Add broth and milk and simmer, uncovered, 10–15 minutes more.

TURKEY SAUSAGE SOUP WITH BEANS AND GREENS

Turkey or chicken sausage is very flavorful and has little of the saturated fat of pork sausage.

12–16 ounces organic mild turkey sausage, cut into cubes
1 tablespoon olive or canola oil
One 15½-ounce can no-salt-added white kidney beans (cannellini), drained and rinsed, or 1½ cups cooked
1 teaspoon oregano
4 cups vegetable or chicken broth (see pages 131–132)
1 pound greens (spinach, kale, or escarole), rinsed and chopped

In a 2-quart pot brown the sausage in the oil. Add the beans, oregano, and broth. Bring to a boil, cover, reduce heat, and simmer for 20 minutes. Meanwhile, in a large pot bring 8 cups of water to a boil and add the greens. Cook for 10 minutes. Drain and chop. Add the cooked greens to the soup and stir.

QUICK-COOKING CHILI

This can be ready to eat in just 30 minutes.

½ cup broth (see page 131)
1 onion, chopped
1 large carrot, peeled and diced
1 clove garlic, minced
2 teaspoons mild chili powder
1 teaspoon ground cumin
One 28-ounce can diced tomatoes
One 15½-ounce can kidney beans or cannellini, drained and rinsed

½ cup bulgur (brown rice or barley can also be substituted)
1 bay leaf

In a large pot heat the broth, add the onion, carrot, and garlic, and cook for 5 minutes or until the carrot and onion are soft. Add all remaining ingredients, stir, and simmer, covered, for 25 minutes or until thickened. Serve by itself or on top of cooked rice or noodles.

HAMBURGER SOUP

This was a family favorite when I was a kid. My children loved it when they were little, too—and they still do.

1 tablespoon olive or canola oil
1 small onion, minced
1 pound ground beef (or ground turkey)
2 small potatoes, peeled and cut into ½-inch pieces
1 carrot, chopped (about 1 cup)
3 cups vegetable broth (see page 132)
1 bay leaf
⅛ teaspoon black pepper (optional)
One 28-ounce can diced tomatoes

In a 2-quart saucepan heat the oil and sauté the onion for 2 minutes. Add beef and brown, breaking up any large lumps and draining excess fat if there is any. Add the potatoes, carrot, broth, bay leaf, and pepper. Bring to a boil, reduce heat, and simmer, covered, for 20 minutes or until potatoes are tender. Stir in tomatoes and cook 10 minutes more, uncovered.

Vegetarian Hamburger Soup: Instead of ground beef use frozen Morningstar Farms veggie crumbles, available in most supermarkets, or 1 cup textured vegetable protein (TVP), sold in health food stores. If using TVP you will need to add an extra cup of broth.

Buying Whole Grains

Wheat, rice, corn, oats, and barley are grains you have already cooked with or at least heard of. In addition, there are many less familiar but delicious and interesting grains to try. The best selections are often in natural food stores, where they are sold by the pound and are often inexpensive. Bulgur, couscous, wheat berries, and quinoa are just a few of the many grains I recommend you try just for the fun of it. Read about whole grains on page 110.

EVERYDAY BEEF, LAMB, AND PORK

MEATBALLS

Meatballs are a convenient way to serve meat to young children. They come in small portions, they are easy to mash, and they are usually served with a tomato-based sauce—a great way to add a serving of vegetables to the menu. This recipe adds grated carrots to the mix for extra flavor and nutrition.

1 cup finely grated zucchini or carrot
1 pound ground beef (or ground turkey)
1 tablespoon finely minced flat parsley
1 clove garlic, chopped fine (optional)
2 eggs
½ cup fresh breadcrumbs, or ¼ cup breadcrumbs and ¼ cup rolled oats

Preheat oven to 375°F. Squeeze the zucchini to remove excess juice. In a bowl combine all ingredients with a spoon or your hands until very well blended. Add more breadcrumbs if the mixture is too wet. Roll mixture between your hands to make 16 mini meatballs. Place the meatballs on a lightly oiled baking sheet. Bake 20 minutes, until meatballs are cooked through and lightly browned. Turn the meatballs at least once while cooking to ensure even browning. Serve with Quick Tomato Sauce (page 169).

Meatloaf: Preheat oven to 350°F. Shape the meat mixture into a loaf and bake on a baking sheet or in a loaf pan 45–60 minutes, until cooked through. Tuck quartered potatoes and quartered onions into the edges of the pan so they can bake with the meat.

MEDITERRANEAN LAMB STEW

As children my daughters loved lamb. This is one of my favorite dishes, too, because you can put it together and let it cook unattended. It also tastes even better the next day. This is delicious served with cooked orzo, or you can add potatoes cut into ½-inch cubes at the same time the green beans are added. Just cook long enough so the potatoes are tender.

1 tablespoon olive oil
1 pound boneless lamb, trimmed of all fat and cut into ½-inch pieces
1 onion, chopped
2 garlic cloves, minced
One 28-ounce can diced tomatoes
1 tablespoon chopped flat parsley
1 bay leaf
One 15½-ounce can chickpeas, drained and rinsed, or 1 ½ cups cooked chickpeas
1 pound green beans, trimmed and chopped into 1-inch pieces

Preheat oven to 350°F. In a Dutch oven heat oil, add lamb pieces, and brown on all sides, about 5 minutes. With a slotted spoon remove lamb and set aside in a bowl. Add onion and cook 5 minutes. Add garlic and cook 2 minutes more. Add tomatoes, parsley, bay leaf, chickpeas, and reserved lamb. Bake, covered, for 30 minutes. Add green beans and cook 15 minutes more, stirring at least once.

POT ROAST

The key to a good pot roast is allowing enough time for it to cook. I have found 3 hours is the right amount of time to guarantee tenderness. Since this is largely unattended cooking, it's almost effortless. Add carrots and potatoes to the pan in the last half hour of cooking and you have a complete one-dish meal good enough for company and perfect for pureeing, mashing, or chopping for the little ones in the house. *For young children:* Serve pieces of meat that have been trimmed of fat, and include some of the cooked vegetables. Gravy is not a nutrition powerhouse, and you don't need to add it for children unless the meat needs a little liquid for mashing or chopping.

¼ cup all-purpose flour plus 2 heaping tablespoons
½ teaspoon garlic powder
1 chuck or rump roast, about 3–4 pounds
1 tablespoon canola oil
2 cups beef or vegetable broth (or use 2 cups water, 3 carrots, diced, 1 onion, quartered, and 1 clove garlic, crushed) plus more as needed for gravy
1 bay leaf
Salt and pepper, or Gravy Master

Preheat oven to 350°F. Put ¼ cup flour and garlic powder in a gallon-size plastic food storage bag and mix well. Add the beef to the bag and toss with the flour so all sides are coated. Remove the beef from the bag and shake off excess flour. Heat the oil in a Dutch oven and brown beef on all sides. Add the broth and bay leaf to the pot, place in the oven, and cook, covered, for 3 hours. Turn the beef once partway through. Add more broth or water if it looks dry. When done, remove the meat from the pan and cover with foil to keep warm while you make the gravy.

With a spoon remove as much fat as you can from the liquid in the pan. Measure remaining liquid and add broth or water to equal 1 cup. In a separate bowl combine the 2 heaping tablespoons of flour with ¼ cup water. Mix into a smooth paste. With the pan over medium heat on the stovetop, whisk half of the flour paste into the liquid. Stir, scraping up browned bits. Add more flour paste until the gravy reaches the desired thickness. Remove the portion to be served to young children and season the remaining gravy with salt and pepper or Gravy Master.

PORK TENDERLOIN

Pork tenderloin is small and cooks quickly. It is very lean, which makes it a good protein choice, but the lack of fat means it can be less tasty and it can dry out quickly. I coat the tenderloin with a blend of mustard and fruit jam to seal in flavor. Because this cut is so lean, you will get no gravy. You can make an interesting sauce by combining ¼ cup of the same jam used in the coating with 1 tablespoon good horseradish. Warm this mixture on the stovetop and serve as a spicy addition to the adult table. Horseradish is too spicy for babies and most toddlers; serve them the pork with warm applesauce instead.

2 tablespoons blueberry or seedless raspberry jam
1 teaspoon mild, smooth mustard
One pork tenderloin, 1–2 pounds
2 apples, cored and quartered
1 large onion, sliced thin

Preheat oven to 375°F. Mix the jam and the mustard and coat the tenderloin with the mixture. Place pork in a nonstick or lightly oiled pan. Tuck the apples and onion under the pork. Roast for 35 minutes or until meat is tender and an instant-read thermometer inserted into the center reads 160°F.

FAMILY BEEF STEW

I love beef stew because once it is assembled it cooks on its own with little attention and everyone loves it. Add dumplings before serving and I think you will find everyone is happy. *For young children:* If your child does not like the dumplings in the stew, remove pieces of meat and vegetables before you add the dumplings, then serve a dumpling on the side like a moist biscuit.

¼ cup all-purpose flour
1½–2 pounds beef chuck, trimmed of fat and cut into 1-inch cubes
1 tablespoon canola oil
1 onion, chopped
3 cups beef or vegetable broth (see pages 132–133)
4 medium potatoes, scrubbed and quartered
4 large carrots, peeled, sliced in half, and cut into ½-inch chunks
1 cup peas, fresh or frozen

Place the flour in a gallon-size plastic food storage bag. Add beef and shake to coat all the pieces. Heat the oil in a stew pot or Dutch oven, add beef, and brown on all sides, cooking in batches if necessary. Add onion and broth, bring to a boil, then reduce heat and simmer, covered, for 45 minutes. Add the potatoes and carrots and cook 25–30 minutes more, or until vegetables are tender. Stir in peas. Remove from heat while you prepare the dumplings.

DUMPLINGS

1 cup all-purpose flour
2 teaspoons baking powder
1 egg
½ cup milk

Mix the flour and baking powder in a bowl. In a separate bowl beat the egg into the milk. Pour the milk mixture over the flour mixture and blend until smooth. Do not overmix. With a spoon, drop the dumpling batter onto the hot stew. Cover, return the stew to the heat, and cook 10 minutes, until dumplings are dry and fluffy.

STUFFED CABBAGE

Young children can be served the inside "stuffing" with the cabbage chopped on the side.

8 large cabbage leaves
1 small onion, finely chopped (about ⅓ cup)
1 tablespoon olive or canola oil
2 cloves garlic, minced
1½ pounds ground beef
½ teaspoon salt
½ teaspoon oregano
¼ teaspoon ground allspice
1 teaspoon paprika (optional)
1 cup cooked brown rice
⅓ cup plain yogurt
1 egg
½ cup breadcrumbs
Quick Tomato Sauce (page 169) or a 15-ounce can of prepared tomato
    sauce (not spaghetti sauce)

Bring a large pot of water to a boil, drop the cabbage leaves in, and cook for 3 minutes. Remove and drain in a colander. In a saucepan cook the onion in the oil for 3 minutes or until soft. Add the garlic, meat, and salt and cook until the meat is no longer pink. Add the oregano, allspice, and paprika and cook 3 minutes more. Remove from heat and stir in the rice and yogurt. Let cool, then mix in the egg and breadcrumbs.

Preheat the oven to 350°F. Remove excess water from the cabbage leaves by blotting them with a paper towel. Place about ½ cup meat mixture on each cabbage leaf and roll. Fold into a package and place seam side down in a lightly oiled pan. Cover with tomato sauce and bake 1 hour.

TACOS

Tacos can be a delicious and healthful combination of meats and vegetables, but don't serve the super-high-sodium seasoning mixes to your family—buy ground cumin and chili powder and make your own. For everyday meals I recommend you skip the cheese or at least use it sparingly because it contains a lot of saturated fat and the meat provides plenty of protein all by itself. Adults who want more heat in their taco can add Tabasco sauce at the table as well as salt and pepper.

1 small onion, finely chopped
1 tablespoon canola oil
1 clove garlic, minced
1 teaspoon ground cumin
¼ teaspoon oregano
2 teaspoons mild chili powder
1 pound ground beef (or ground turkey)
Juice of 1 lime
¼ teaspoon salt
8 soft tortillas or 6 small taco shells*
1 cup chopped tomatoes
1 cucumber, chopped
1 cup shredded lettuce
½ cup whole-milk yogurt or sour cream
Salsa
Shredded cheese (optional)

In a saucepan sauté the onion in the oil until soft, about 5 minutes. Add garlic, cook 1 minute, then add cumin, oregano, chili powder, and ground beef. Cook over medium heat until beef is no longer pink, breaking up lumps. Stir in lime juice and salt. Taste and correct seasonings. Preheat the oven to 350°F. Wrap the soft tortillas in foil and heat 5 minutes. Place the hard tacos on a baking pan and heat 5 minutes. Assemble the remaining ingredients on a platter and serve with the cooked meat, allowing everyone to build their version of the perfect taco.

*For young children do not use crisp taco shells, as they can be a choking hazard.

STUFFED PEPPERS

If you want to experiment with whole grains, try brown rice. If you are in a hurry, use Uncle Ben's Ready Rice brown rice.

This is a very easy way to add whole grains to your menu. *For young children:* A whole pepper is way too big for most little ones. Scoop out some of the filling, chop some of the pepper, and serve them together.

4 whole peppers
1 small onion, finely chopped
1 tablespoon canola oil
½ pound ground beef
One 14-ounce can diced tomatoes, drained
2 eggs, beaten
1 cup cooked rice
¼ cup grated cheddar or Monterey jack cheese

Cut the top off each pepper and scrape out the seeds. Plunge the peppers into a pot of boiling water and parboil until just tender, about 3 minutes. Remove with a slotted spoon and rinse with cold water. In a skillet cook the onion in the oil until tender, about 3 minutes. Add beef, breaking up lumps. Cook until meat is no longer pink. Remove from heat and stir in tomatoes, eggs, and rice. Return to heat and cook until egg is set. The mixture should be moist but not soupy. Remove from heat, stir in cheese, and let cool before stuffing peppers. Fill the peppers with the mixture. Place in a baking dish and bake in a preheated 375°F oven for 20 minutes. Serve with Quick Tomato Sauce (page 169).

EVERYDAY FISH

Fish is truly a health food, but many people do not know how to cook it. Buy fish fresh when you can, but frozen fish is a very good and often less expensive alternative.

BAKED FISH

This is a universal fish recipe for any fish fillet. The key to this recipe is a hot oven. *For young children:* A fillet should be free of all bones, but always check before serving to a very young child.

1 pound fish fillets
¼ cup breadcrumbs
¼ teaspoon dried oregano
1 tablespoon olive oil
Lemon wedges

Preheat oven to 450°F. Place a rack in the top third of the oven. Place fish fillets in a lightly oiled ovenproof dish. Combine bread crumbs, oregano, and oil and sprinkle evenly over fish. Bake 7 to 10 minutes. Fish is cooked when it loses its translucency and flakes easily. You can also use an instant-read thermometer; fish is done at a temperature of 140°F. Serve with lemon wedges.

BROILED WILD-CAUGHT SALMON

Salmon is an almost unbeatable source of the fatty acid DHA. When wild salmon is available, buy several pieces and freeze it; it keeps well for 4–6 weeks.

1 pound wild-caught salmon fillet

Preheat broiler. Place the fish on a lightly oiled roasting pan. Broil 3 inches from the heat for 5–6 minutes for a fillet ¾ to 1 inch thick. Thicker pieces will take a little longer.

FISH WITH PASTA

This was one of our family favorites when the children were younger because the pasta was so popular with the kids and the fish was popular with me. Serve with a vegetable—I like it with peas or green beans. *For young children:* Always check for bones even when using a fillet.

1 clove garlic, minced
2 tablespoons olive oil

*1 pound white fish (such as haddock, monkfish, or cod), cut into
   2-inch chunks*
½ cup fish, clam, or vegetable broth
¼ cup water
1 tablespoon chopped fresh basil (or flat parsley or cilantro)
¼ teaspoon dried oregano
½ pound pasta
Lemon wedges (optional)
Grated parmesan cheese (optional)

In a 2-quart saucepan sauté the garlic in the oil for 1 minute.
Add fish, broth, water, basil, and oregano. Cover and simmer
for 10 minutes. While the fish simmers, cook the pasta according to package instructions. Remove fish from heat and stir
gently so as not to break up the fish too much. Drain the
pasta, put it in a large bowl, and pour all of the fish with its
cooking liquid over the pasta. Add a squeeze of lemon juice
and toss with grated cheese.

EVERYDAY POULTRY

Children enjoy chicken, and it is a delicious source of lean protein
and minerals, too.

ROAST CHICKEN

1 whole chicken, 3–4 pounds
2 tablespoons olive oil or melted butter
Garlic powder or fresh minced garlic

Preheat the oven to 375°F. Rinse chicken, pat dry, and place in
a roasting pan. Rub the chicken with the oil or butter and
sprinkle with garlic powder or fresh garlic, rubbing so it is
evenly distributed. Cook 20 minutes per pound. Insert a thermometer into the thickest part of the thigh, making sure it
does not touch the bone. It will read 160–165°F when the
chicken is done.

Roast Chicken with Vegetables: Cut 4 baking potatoes in half, place in the roasting pan along with 4–6 peeled whole carrots and 2 whole onions, peeled, before you put the pan in the oven. They will roast in the juices and be yummy.

Gravy: If you want a little more flavor, add a whole peeled garlic clove to the pan with chicken before you put it in the oven. It will become very soft and blend easily into the drippings. Have ready ¼ cup flour and 1–1½ cups chicken broth. Remove the chicken and vegetables from the pan. Pour the drippings into a bowl and skim off the fat. Combine about ¼ cup of the fat with the flour to make a paste. Return the drippings to the roasting pan and place on the stovetop. Add the flour mixture and cook over low heat until the mixture is smooth and thick. Add enough broth to thin the gravy to the consistency you like.

BAKED CHICKEN

You can use chicken breasts, but I recommend chicken thighs for this dish because they are more flavorful and less expensive.

1 pound boneless, skinless chicken breast, cut into 4 pieces, or 1 pound boneless, skinless chicken thighs (4 pieces)
¼ cup mustard
Breadcrumbs made from 2 English muffins, or 1 cup plain breadcrumbs

Preheat oven to 350°F. Lightly oil a casserole dish. Place the chicken in a gallon-size plastic food storage bag, add the mustard, and toss until each piece is covered. Place the breadcrumbs in another plastic bag and add one piece of chicken at a time, coating with the crumbs. Place chicken in the pan and bake 20–30 minutes, until chicken is cooked and crumbs are lightly browned.

Does This Exchange Sound Familiar?

SIX-YEAR-OLD CHILD, looking at a plate of homemade maca-
roni and cheese: "What's that?"
GRANDMOTHER: "Macaroni and cheese."
CHILD: "Ours is orange and comes out of a box."

EVERYDAY VEGETARIAN MEALS

MACARONI AND CHEESE

I have to admit my mother served me macaroni and cheese
out of a box, and I turned to the boxed version, too, when in
a rush or traveling. I include this recipe because it is a popular
meatless meal, and if you serve it with a sliced fruit or a vegetable on the side, it makes a nice dinner for everyone.

3 tablespoons butter
3 tablespoons all-purpose flour
3½ cups milk★
1½ cups grated cheddar cheese
½ cup grated parmesan cheese
1 teaspoon Dijon mustard (optional)
1 pound elbow macaroni or ziti, white or whole-wheat
½–1 cup plain breadcrumbs
1 tablespoon olive oil

Preheat the oven to 375°F. Oil a 9-by-13-inch pan. Melt the
butter in a medium-size saucepan, stir in flour, and cook for
2–3 minutes. Slowly pour in 1 cup of the milk and stir or
whisk until smooth. Add remaining milk and bring almost to
a boil. Lower heat and simmer for 3 minutes. Stir in cheeses
and mustard. Turn off heat and set aside.

★Children under two years of age are to be served whole milk as a beverage because they need the fat calories. In this dish cheese provides
plenty of calories, so making use of skim, 1 percent, or 2 percent milk
is a good idea.

Cook the pasta as directed on the package. Drain. Combine cheese sauce and pasta and pour into prepared pan. Combine breadcrumbs with olive oil and sprinkle over pasta. Bake 30–40 minutes, until the cheese is bubbly and the crumbs brown. Can be assembled ahead, covered, and kept refrigerated for 1 day before baking.

QUICK TOMATO SAUCE

This is a simple recipe. If you prefer a smooth sauce, remove the bay leaf and puree sauce in the blender or food processor. Strain if needed. Freeze small portions in an ice cube tray.

MAKES ABOUT 4 CUPS SAUCE

1 small onion, finely chopped
2 tablespoons olive oil
1 clove garlic, minced
One 28-ounce can diced no-salt-added tomatoes
One 28-ounce can crushed tomatoes
1 bay leaf
2 tablespoons capers (optional)
2 tablespoons chopped pitted black olives, preferably oil-cured or Greek (optional)

In a medium-size saucepan cook the onion in the oil until soft, about 5 minutes. Add garlic and cook 1 minute more. Add all remaining ingredients. Bring to a boil, reduce heat, cover, and simmer 20 minutes.

LAZY VEGETABLE LASAGNA

This can be assembled in 10 minutes and tastes fabulous. Until the vegetables thaw the dish will look lumpy and uneven, but don't worry—as it heats up all the ingredients will blend together.

1 pound ricotta, low-fat or regular
1 cup grated mozzarella
1 egg

1 pound frozen Italian-style vegetables
One 28-ounce can diced tomatoes, drained
½ teaspoon oregano
One 26-ounce jar spaghetti sauce
8 no-bake lasagna noodles
½ cup parmesan

Preheat oven to 350°F. Lightly oil a lasagna pan. In a large bowl combine the ricotta and mozzarella; add egg and combine well. Fold in the frozen vegetables, tomatoes, and oregano.

Spread ½ cup spaghetti sauce on the bottom of the lasagna pan and cover the bottom with four lasagna noodles. Spoon half the cheese-vegetable mixture over the noodles and spread evenly. Top with ½ cup sauce and repeat with four more noodles and the remaining cheese-vegetable mixture. Top with the remaining sauce. Sprinkle with parmesan, cover with aluminum foil, and bake 30 minutes. Uncover and bake 10 minutes more. Allow to rest a few minutes before serving.

POLENTA WITH CHEESE AND ROASTED VEGETABLES

4 cups water
1 cup cornmeal
Salt
½ cup prepared tomato sauce
1 cup ricotta
2 cups roasted vegetables (see page 171) (onion, carrots, and red
  peppers are a good combination)
2 tablespoons parmesan

Bring water to a boil, add cornmeal and a pinch of salt, and cook, stirring, until smooth. Preheat oven to 375°F. Lightly oil a lasagna pan. Spread the polenta evenly in the pan. Top evenly with the sauce, then the ricotta. Add the roasted vegetable and sprinkle with the parmesan. Bake for 20 minutes.

Vegetable Cooking Primer

To steam vegetables: Set a steamer basket or collapsible metal steamer insert inside a pan and add an inch or so of water. Put the vegetables in the basket, bring the water to a boil, cover, and cook 2–5 minutes, depending on how big the vegetable pieces are. If you do not have a steamer, place chopped vegetables in an inch of water, cover, and steam until tender. Vegetables are done when you can pierce them with a fork.

To roast vegetables: Cut vegetables into same-size pieces. Asparagus, beets, carrots, eggplant, parsnips, peppers, winter squash, and onions are just a few possibilities. Toss with a little oil and spread in a single layer on a baking sheet. Roast at 400°F for 20 minutes or until tender, turning once.

EVERYDAY DESSERT

A fruit-based dessert is one of my favorite ways to satisfy a sweet tooth. It tastes good and is good for you, too.

POACHED FRUIT

Pears, peaches, apricots, and even figs are delicious poached and served warm with a dollop of good yogurt, whipped cream, or ice cream. I usually leave the skins on, but they can be removed before cooking if you prefer. For an extra treat drizzle with a prepared hot fudge sauce or caramel sauce before serving.

1 cup orange juice (or peach-flavored grape juice)
1 teaspoon vanilla
1 stick cinnamon (optional; omit if using peach-flavored grape juice)
4 pears or peaches, or 6–8 apricots or fresh figs, cored and cut in half

In a 4-quart saucepan combine the juice, vanilla, and cinnamon. Add the fruit cut side down and simmer, covered, for

20–30 minutes. Remove fruit and set aside. Raise the heat and simmer the juices until they reduce to about ½ cup. Pour over the fruit.

BAKED APPLES

This is so simple it barely needs a recipe. Core as many apples as you want to cook. Sprinkle with cinnamon. Place in an oven-safe dish and bake at 350°F for 30 minutes. Or microwave for 1 minute for 1 apple.

APPLE CRISP

This is traditionally made with apples, but peaches and blueberries can replace the apples. Or combine different fruits to make a unique dessert.

4 cups apples, peeled, cored, and sliced
½ cup rolled oats
¼ cup all-purpose flour
½ cup packed brown sugar
½ stick butter, softened
1 teaspoon cinnamon
¼ teaspoon freshly grated nutmeg (optional)

Preheat oven to 350°F. Place the fruit in a 9-inch pie plate or casserole. In a small bowl combine all remaining ingredients and with fingertips blend the ingredients until crumbly. Sprinkle over the fruit. Bake 30 minutes.

FRUIT COBBLER

Made with blueberries and apples and with cornmeal in the topping, this is superb.

4 cups cored, seeded, chopped fresh fruit (apples, blueberries,
    nectarines, peaches, pears, plums, or a combination), skins left on
1¼ cups sugar

¼ teaspoon cinnamon

1 tablespoon instant tapioca

1 tablespoon unsalted butter, firm, plus 4 tablespoons unsalted butter,
    softened

1½ cups all-purpose flour, or a combination of whole-grain flours
    (even cornmeal and ground flaxseed)

2½ teaspoons baking powder

½ cup milk

Preheat oven to 350°F and grease an 8-inch round casserole. Toss the fruit with ¾ cup sugar, cinnamon, and tapioca. Pour into prepared dish and dot with 1 tablespoon firm butter. Combine the flour, ½ cup sugar, and baking powder, and with clean fingers blend 4 tablespoons softened butter into the flour until no visible pieces remain. Stir in the milk to make a thick batter and pour over the fruit. Bake 30 minutes until brown on top and fruit bubbles.

CHERRI CLAFOUTI

This is a lot like a cobbler, only the batter is made with eggs.

1 pound cherries, pits removed, or other fruit such as 4 cups
    blueberries or peeled, chopped apples, pears, or peaches

1 cup flour

¾ cup sugar

4 eggs

1½ cup milk

Preheat oven to 350°F. Layer the fruit in an oiled 8-inch round casserole. Mix flour and sugar. Beat eggs with milk, then pour ½ cup milk mixture over the flour and combine. Gradually stir in the rest of the milk mixture. Pour batter over the fruit and bake 40 to 50 minutes.

Parchment Paper

Keep a supply of parchment paper on hand and use it to line cookie sheets. It practically eliminates cleanup, increasing the chances you will do more baking.

FREE-FORM FRUIT TART

Master this dessert and you can have a yummy fruit dessert ready quickly using seasonal fruits. The cookie crumbs absorb the juices.

1 prepared pie crust for a 9-inch pie
1 tablespoon brown or white sugar
½ cup crushed vanilla cookie or graham cracker crumbs
2 apples, peeled, cored, and sliced thin
1 tablespoon lemon juice
1 tablespoon jam, your favorite flavor

Preheat oven to 400°F. On a floured board roll out the pastry until it is about 12 inches in diameter. Transfer the dough to a parchment paper–lined cookie sheet. Sprinkle dough with the sugar and cookie crumbs. Toss the apples with the lemon juice and spread in the crust (you can make a nice design if you have the time). Leave a 1–2-inch border without fruit or crumbs. Heat the jam in the microwave until it liquefies, about 45 seconds, and spread over the fruit using a pastry brush. Lift the edges of the dough to cover the fruit. Bake 20 minutes.

Variation: Instead of apples, substitute 2 cups sliced plums or peaches. Berries can be used, too. Combine 2 cups chopped strawberries, blueberries, or raspberries or any combination with 1 tablespoon instant tapioca or 1 tablespoon cornstarch, and omit the jam glaze. If using rhubarb, you will need to add 1 cup sugar.

PUMPKIN CAKE

Buy whole nutmeg and grate it fresh each time you need some; the flavor is much better than preground nutmeg.

1 cup all-purpose flour (or half whole-wheat and half all-purpose)
½ teaspoon cinnamon
2 teaspoons baking powder
¼ teaspoon salt
½ teaspoon freshly ground nutmeg
½ teaspoon ground cloves
½ teaspoon ground ginger
1 cup sugar
One 15-ounce can pure pumpkin (not pie filling)
½ cup canola oil
¾–1 cup plain yogurt
2 eggs

Preheat oven to 350°F. Grease an 8-inch square pan. In a large bowl thoroughly combine flour, cinnamon, baking powder, salt, nutmeg, cloves, ginger, and sugar. Make a well in the flour mixture and add the pumpkin, oil, yogurt, and eggs. Mix until moistened, but do not overmix. Pour into pan and bake 35–40 minutes. Cake is done when a knife inserted into the center comes out clean. Cool in the pan on a rack for 10 minutes, then remove from pan and cool completely.

BLUEBERRY CAKE

1¾ cups plus 1 tablespoon sugar
1 stick butter, softened
1 teaspoon vanilla or 1 teaspoon lemon extract
¾ cup plain yogurt
2 eggs
1½ cups all-purpose flour
1½ teaspoons baking powder
¼ teaspoon salt

2 cups fresh or frozen blueberries
2 teaspoons cinnamon

Preheat oven to 350°F. Coat an 8-inch springform pan with cooking spray and sprinkle with 1 tablespoon sugar to cover sides. In a bowl beat together 1½ cups sugar and butter until light and fluffy, 2–3 minutes. Add vanilla, yogurt, and eggs and mix well. In another bowl combine flour, baking powder, and salt. Add to yogurt mixture. Combine the cinnamon and ¼ cup sugar. Set half of the cinnamon-sugar mixture aside and toss blueberries with the remaining cinnamon sugar. Fold sugared berries gently into the batter. Pour the batter into the pan and sprinkle with the reserved cinnamon-sugar mixture. Bake for 1 hour. Cake is done when a knife inserted into the center comes out clean. Cool in the pan on a rack at least 15 minutes, then remove sides of pan and cool completely.

Apple Cake: Replace the blueberries with 3 cups chopped peeled apples.

OATMEAL COOKIES

I love homemade oatmeal cookies. For a change of pace I mix in ½ cup chocolate chips or raisins.

MAKES 24 COOKIES

1 stick butter, softened
⅓ cup packed brown sugar
⅓ cup granulated sugar
1 egg
1 teaspoon vanilla
½ cup white whole-wheat flour
½ cup all-purpose flour
1 teaspoon baking powder
1 cup rolled oats

Preheat oven to 350°F. Cream the butter with the sugars until light and fluffy. Beat in the egg and vanilla. Blend in the remaining dry ingredients. Drop by tablespoonfuls on a parchment-lined or greased cookie sheet and bake 10 minutes, until lightly browned.

Batch Cooking

Cooking extra portions will save you time and money. There is nothing more satisfying than turning to your freezer for a delicious homemade casserole when you are too tired to cook. One good friend of mine was given a baby shower for her second child and instead of gifts, everyone was asked to bring a dish she could store in her freezer until after the baby came. She loved it.

To make batch cooking effective, keep these points in mind:

- Label everything. Include the name of the food, the date you made it, and cooking instructions if needed.
- Use the right freezer products, such as plastic containers and resealable bags.
- Cool food before freezing so you don't put a strain on your freezer.
- Freeze in portions that are practical. You may want to make a big pot of stew, for example, but freeze it in single portions.

The Well-Stocked Kitchen

I have had so many parents tell me they end up eating pizza, sub sandwiches, or even ice cream for dinner because they were starving and had nothing in the house to cook. Don't let that become a habit for you. Use this list to evaluate what you have and replenish what you need. I suggest you always have the ingredients on hand to make a simple breakfast, lunch, and dinner. Keeping cupboards, refrigerators, and freezers stocked with good food and the ingredients to make a quick meal is one of the best strategies for eating well in today's world.

When you shop for fresh foods, buy only what you will cook within the week or can freeze. In general, shop for fresh items when you will have the most time to cook. For example, if you work Monday through Friday, shop on Thursday so you have the weekend to cook, eat, and enjoy fresh foods. This way food won't go bad because you did not have time to cook it.

Cans/Jars/Boxes

Tomatoes: canned tomatoes, tomato sauce, tomato paste
Canned beans: chickpeas, cannellini, kidney beans
Canned fish: tuna, salmon
Low-sodium broth
Prepared soup
No-salt-added vegetables
Canned fruit (in juice or light syrup)
Cereal, hot and cold
Flour: white, whole-wheat, other
Grains: brown and white rice, barley
Pasta: spaghetti, no-boil lasagna, orzo, egg noodles
Crackers: graham, animal, teething biscuits, flatbread, Fig Newtons, gingersnaps
Popcorn
Nuts for eating, peanut butter
Coffee, tea, bottled water and seltzer, bottled juice

Frozen

Freeze meat in meal-size portions, usually not more than 1 pound

Fish fillet or shrimp
Beef for stew or ground beef

Chicken or turkey breast or skinless thighs
Veggie burgers
Fruit juice concentrate
Whole unsweetened fruit (pineapple, blueberries, raspberries, strawberries)
Vegetables (peas, spinach, corn)
Burritos
Pierogis
Ravioli or tortellini
Frozen desserts: sherbet, ice cream
Nuts for baking

Fats/Oils

Olive oil
Canola oil
Salad dressing
Mayonnaise
Butter
Soft margarine

Seasonings/Dry Goods

Bay leaves
Cinnamon
Chili powder
Cumin
Oregano
Nutmeg
Salt
Pepper
Honey
Maple syrup
Jams
Ketchup
Mustard

Fresh Foods

Eggs
Fruit
Lemons
Vegetables (onion, garlic, potato)
Beef
Chicken
Pork
Fish
Dairy (milk, cheese, yogurt, butter)
Bread: whole-wheat, white, rye, pita, tortillas, wraps, English
  muffins (if family members have different bread prefer-
  ences, buy what everyone wants and freeze what will not be
  used right away; it can be thawed quickly)

High-Fructose Corn Syrup

High-fructose corn syrup (HFCS) was invented in 1960. It is made by processing cornstarch to yield glucose (a form of sugar), then processing the glucose into a syrup with a very high percentage of another form of sugar called fructose. HFCS is relatively cheap, which is why it is now the dominant sweetener in our food and drinks—between 1970 and 1990 per capita consumption increased 1,000 percent.

Many nutritionists have concerns that HFCS is metabolized differently than regular table sugar and might be the cause of our national rise in obesity and diabetes. This is an unproven concern; it is the impact HCFS has on this generation's perception of sweetness that worries me. Many of the commercial granola bars, crackers, and baked goods you will want to feed your child are made with HFCS. These products will always be sweeter than your homemade versions and for that reason can easily become your child's preferred choice. I fear that the child who develops a preference for HFCS-sweetened food early in life may be prone to overeat because he craves the intense sweetness in these foods and the products usually made with HFCS rarely include fruit, fiber, or whole grains, ingredients that lead to satiety.

Eating Advice for Harried Parents

This is a baby food book, but there is nothing more important to a child's well-being than a healthy mom or dad. Right now you are shaping the routines that will impact how much weight you gain over the next twenty years. Eating too much at night, snacking on the wrong foods, drinking high-calorie beverages, not eating enough fruits and vegetables, and not finding the time to exercise are the reasons so many adults steadily gain weight. Here is some advice to start practicing now to prevent creeping weight gain.

Late-night eating. If you want to enjoy a treat once the baby is in bed, limit portion size. Have one piece of chocolate or one serving of low-fat ice cream—calories count!

Between-meal snacks. Select foods that improve your health but don't lead to overeating. I recommend fruit of any kind, yogurt, or vegetables. If you choose chips or crackers, limit them to a 100-calorie portion.

Fruits and vegetables. Eat a fruit or vegetable (or both) at every meal. At lunch and supper fill half your plate with vegetables.

Beverages. The best choices are water, black coffee, and tea. Limit any soda, diet or regular, to one per day. If you drink juice, have only 6 ounces per day. Though milk is a good food, two to three 8-ounce servings is all any adult needs.

Movement. Keep trying to find time for exercise. It is good for your body and sense of well-being, and it makes you a good role model for your child.

Cooking with Sugar

I cook with sugar because it is an honest sweetener. We all know sugar has no vitamins or minerals, but it has been in use for centuries with no side effects that cannot be controlled with tooth brushing and portion control. I use brown sugar and honey in recipes when I want a slightly different taste— both honey and brown sugar carry only trace amounts of nutrients. White sugar can be replaced by an equal amount of packed brown sugar in most recipes. To use honey instead of sugar, some of the liquid must be reduced. Use the following formula: 2 tablespoons sugar can be replaced by 3 tablespoons honey and reduce the liquid in the recipe by 2 tablespoons.

All artificial sweeteners are to be avoided when cooking for children because they offer no calories or nutrition and because of potential side effects that may include behavior changes, headaches, and even an increased risk of cancer. Better to serve real sugar in small amounts. The only exception to this would be the child with diabetes. If you have family members who cook with artificial sweeteners, one bite won't harm your child. It is the accumulated dose over time that concerns me.

Fruit: Is It Too High in Sugar for Babies?

Parents who follow diets that restrict carbohydrates or who avoid foods with a high glycemic index often tell me they worry about serving their children fruit because they fear it will cause obesity or alter blood sugar levels. Fruit may have a relatively high glycemic index, but unlike white sugar the carbohydrate in fruit is accompanied by fiber, vitamins, minerals, and antioxidants. Children who eat fruit consistently have better diets than non-fruit-eaters.

Everybody Loves Pizza

Pizza is not a baby food, of course, but it will be in your child's future because it is so popular. Just one of the top ten frozen pizza companies sells over $800 million worth of pizza each year. Among my clients pizza is consistently identified as a problem food because it is so high in calories. In general I tell families not to serve pizza more than once per week, and only once a month if anyone in the house is trying to lose weight. When ordering a take-out pizza, improve the quality of what you order by asking for less cheese and more vegetables. To serve a healthier pizza at home, choose a 15-ounce frozen cheese pizza that contains about 1,200 calories. Before baking, top it with 1–2 cups of chopped vegetables tossed with a little oil. Cook as directed.

SEVEN

How to Shop

As I said earlier, when it comes to food we have more to think about than previous generations did. Deciding what to eat was not so complex when choices were based on availability, which was dictated by location and the seasons. Now we have choice—lots and lots of choice. As parents, we want to make the right choices. Now add politics to our decision making, and we have even more questions. Should we buy organic, local, Certified Humane, natural, or fortified foods? Is genetically modified food unsafe? What about irradiated food? These are not trivial decisions for your family. What you buy impacts your baby's future in terms of both personal health and the health of the communities we live in.

According to the Economic Policy Institute, a family of four living in my area of southern New Hampshire can expect to budget at least $587 each month for food. That adds up to over $7,000 each year. Those food dollars can impact issues that go beyond nutrition, such as the environment and the humane treatment of animals. Be aware that how you spend your money influences the food world that your child will inherit. You may have heard the expression "voting with your fork." Each time you make a food purchase you tell a company that you want more of the same, and it is time parents start asking for the best foods for ourselves, our children, and the planet.

ORGANIC FOOD

I recommend you buy organic food whenever you can, because it will be better for your baby's health as well as the environment. Organic foods carry no antibiotics or growth hormones and are free of conventional pesticides, synthetic fertilizer, bioengineering, and irradiation. Beginning in 2002, the U.S. Department of Agriculture put in place a national standard for the term "organic." This applies to both domestic and imported food. Foods can be certified "100% organic" if the entire product is organic or "organic" if 95 to 99 percent of the ingredients are organic. A food label can also state "made with organic ingredients" if at least 70 percent of the ingredients are organic. Products made with less than 70 percent organic ingredients can list specific organic ingredients on the side panel but the product cannot make an organic claim on the front of the package. The product look-up (PLU) code, which is the little sticker on fruit and vegetables, identifies organic food by starting with the number 9. The government standards program carries fines for misuse, which means you can trust the organic seal. Additional claims such as "natural," "free-range," or "hormone-free" may be truthful, but those claims are not independently verified and are not to be confused with being organic. "Natural" applied to meat or poultry means the product carries no artificial colors, flavors, or preservatives. "Natural" and "all-natural" when applied to non-meat products are meaningless words with no standard definition. Go to www.ams.usda.gov/nop for additional information about organic food and labeling.

Not everyone can find or afford to eat organic food all the time. So the next question is, when is it important and when is it less important? Take comfort in knowing that food grown and purchased in the United States is probably the safest and healthiest food anywhere in the world, organic or not. Here are my suggestions. Buy organic versions of the produce highest in pesticide residues (see box on page 191). If you peel produce, pesticide residues will be lowered even further. Foods that have a high fat content such as meat, poultry, dairy, and oils should be organic as often as possible because fat holds on to pesticides. When I can't find organic I look for foods grown in the United States and as close to my home as possible. Even non-organic food grown in this country is protected from excessive pesticide levels by the Food Quality Protection Act (FQPA), which requires the Environmental Protection Agency (EPA) to set safety factors that consider the unique vulnerability of children. Buying "local" reduces the cost of commercial food production, and because the food travels less, it will be fresher and richer in nutrients. Read more about local food below.

COUNTRY-OF-ORIGIN LABELING

In 2002 Congress passed a law requiring country-of-origin labeling (COOL) on most foods. You will be most likely to see examples of this in the fish market and in the produce aisle. By 2008, most foods should be labeled with country of origin. I find this particularly helpful in choosing locally grown foods and foods produced in this country.

ARTIFICIAL COLORS AND PRESERVATIVES

Read labels on food and fruit juice and avoid those with added colors or the preservative sodium benzoate. A 2007 study in the *Lancet* found these additives increased hyperactivity in young children.

LOCAL FOOD

Local food is generally defined as food grown within a hundred-mile radius of where it is purchased. The trend in buying and marketing food as "local" has benefits for you as a consumer. Besides providing better taste and nutrition, buying locally can support your local farmers, can increase the diversity of food choices, and could help control climate change by reducing the miles a food travels to be sold. For more information about this movement and where to find farmers' markets, go to www.slowfoodsusa.org.

GENETICALLY MODIFIED FOODS

Genetically modified (GM) foods or genetically modified organism (GMO) foods are also known as bioengineered foods. Food growers choose these techniques to improve production. Plants may be modified to be disease-resistant, produce higher yields, or stay fresh longer without spoiling. Altering foods at the genetic level worries many people. The greatest concern is modifying a food with genes from other species in order to add perceived beneficial qualities and creating an allergy risk that did not exist in the original food. For example, a tomato that is genetically modified to carry a gene from a peanut might make the food intolerable to anyone with a peanut allergy—without that person being aware of the potential risk. Genetically modified foods are not easy to identify. For produce, you can look at the product look-up (PLU) code—GM and GMO foods are to be identified with a PLU code beginning in 8. But other GM foods are not required by law to list that they are GM. Organic foods should be GMO-free.

IRRADIATION

Irradiated foods are supposed to carry the flower-like radura symbol and state that they have been treated with irradiation. Foods may be treated with gamma rays, X-rays, or electron beams intended to kill potentially crop-damaging insects such as fruit flies or bacteria on beef that can cause food poisoning. It is likely that many of the spices you already eat have been irradiated. Irradiated food is not radioactive, but consumers often don't like the idea of irradiated food because they are concerned that it will alter a food's nutritive value. The effect of irradiation on nutrition has not, in fact, been proven, but nutritionists worry about irradiation covering up poor food-handling practices. Irradiation can control food bacteria and spoilage, but keeping processing areas clean and food stored at the right temperature can do the same thing with no risk. The Food and Drug Administration has recently suggested allowing some irradiated foods to be labeled as "pasteurized," as the process kills bacteria. The use of that term will only add to confusion in the marketplace. Irradiated food should be clearly identified so families can make informed choices.

GROWTH HORMONE IN BEEF AND DAIRY CATTLE AND SHEEP

Cattle and sheep may be treated with growth hormones to speed growth. The use of hormones is permitted as long as there are no residues in meat when they arrive in the marketplace. Many consumers are uncomfortable with this. Look for the phrase "No Added Hormones" on beef labels or the organic seal as a way to avoid hormones in meat.

Recombinant bovine somatotropin (rbST) is a hormone given to cows to increase milk production. Users say it is not harmful to our health because it is inactivated and digested in the stomach. Cows treated with rbST are forced to produce more milk than they would naturally, causing physical stress and increasing cases of the bacterial infection called mastitis, which requires the administration of more antibiotics. In New England, where I live, milk from growth-hormone-free cows is plentiful and clearly labeled, and though it costs a bit more, I recommend it. The protein and calcium levels in both products will be the same, but the idea of unnecessarily ingesting growth hormone and forcing animals to overproduce is enough to make me look for the hormone-free products. Milk that has been certified organic is from cows fed an organic diet, and the cows will not be treated with hormones or antibiotics.

CERTIFIED HUMANE

I am not a vegetarian, but I make it a priority to eat meat from animals that at least had a decent life. For that reason I look for food that has "Certified Humane" on the label. It means that meat, poultry, eggs, or dairy products come from animals raised meeting humane standards, including sufficient space and access to fresh water and a good diet. For more information and a list of foods carrying the symbol, go to www.certifiedhumane.com.

THERE IS MORE THAT YOU CAN DO

As I mentioned, today's generation of parents is the key to shaping our future world of food in desirable ways. Since the 1980s our food supply has been altered to meet our demand for good-tasting, inexpensive food. But this has come at a very real cost to many of us. The medical costs of obesity in the United States are estimated to be $100 billion a year. These costs are incurred to treat diabetes, high blood pressure, orthopedic problems, and even cancer associated with obesity. This is a figure that will only go up, and you and your family will be impacted by it even if you yourself are not overweight.

You might think that educating adults and children would help counter this, but in an Associated Press article that examined the impact of fifty-seven nutrition education programs designed to get children to eat better, only four showed any promise in changing the way children eat. Some may have even been counterproductive. In 2007, the article estimated, the federal government would spend more than $1 billion on nutrition education, but based on previous results much of that will have no effect. This is where you come in.

You are your child's most effective teacher, and how you feed your family will make all the difference. The statistics on diet-related disease are unequivocal, and while it seems like the task of getting people to eat better is immensely complex, there is plenty of evidence to suggest that a single dietary change—eating the recommended number of servings of fruits and vegetables—could reverse problematic health trends. The addition of fruits and vegetables to meals reduces intake of calories, sodium, and cholesterol while adding potassium, fiber, and vitamins. This combination lowers blood pressure, blood sugar, and serum cholesterol. It promotes a sense of satiety and can prevent obesity. I recommend that adults fill half their plates with vegetables at both lunch and dinner, eat a serving of whole fruit at breakfast, and include a fruit or vegetable when snacking between meals. Very young children may get too full on low-calorie foods at meals if they eat half their plate as vegetables; offer children a serving of fruit, vegetable, or both at mealtime and include a fruit or vegetable as part of snacks. Practice this style of eating as part of everyday meals and you will be implementing the dietary recommendations that prevent disease.

FOR THE LOVE OF FOOD PROJECT

In the spring of 2007 I started a project called For the Love of Food: teaching friends and family to eat better through small dinner parties and family meals. At these dinner parties a meal is planned and served following two simple principles. First, the menu follows a formula that includes appetizers (or snacks) that are vegetable-based and requires half the dinner plate to be filled with vegetables and dessert to be fruit based. Second, everyone is to have a seat at the table and enjoy the meal, conversation, and company. At the end of the meal the guests are asked to "pass it on" to their friends or family. It is hoped that this project can give the experience of eating a menu that is rich in fruits and vegetables and truly healthful. Through sharing recipes and returning to planned meals, we can reverse the rising trend in obesity and its diet-related diseases. I invite everyone reading this book to participate. Imagine the potential if we all participated in this "chain" dinner party. For menu ideas and instructions on how you, too, can participate, please go to www.fortheloveoffood.org.

RECOMMENDED READING

Three very good books on the subject of our contemporary food environment include *What to Eat* by Marion Nestle, *The Omnivore's Dilemma* by Michael Pollan, and *The Way We Eat: Why Our Food*

Choices Matter by Peter Singer and Jim Mason. I have also found the Whole Foods Market Web page to be a good source of practical food information: www.wholefoodsmarket.com. For an accurate scientific discussion, go to the site of the Center for Science in the Public Interest, www.cspinet.org, and search for the topic that concerns you. Better yet, subscribe to their newsletter, *Nutrition Action Healthletter.*

Suggestions for Controlling Costs

Food cost is an issue for me, and I am sure it is for you, too. The organic foods that have the most sticker shock for me are meat, poultry, eggs, and butter. To control costs I practice portion control and use very little of certain foods, like butter or meat. On one day I could spend $8 on a free-range organic chicken, and the next day I might spend only 69 cents on a can of beans to make a vegetarian stew. When I average the cost of protein between the two meals it comes out to a little over $4, which fits in my budget. This style of eating is also healthier because I am consuming less animal fat and more plant-based foods. I also buy frozen fruit and vegetables. I like them because they are flash frozen, which retains most of their nutrients, and they will last for quite a while if kept frozen.

Foods to Buy Organic:
The Environmental Working Group's "Dirty Dozen"

The conventionally grown produce with the highest pesticide residues include peaches, apples, sweet bell peppers, celery, nectarines, strawberries, cherries, pears, imported grapes, spinach, lettuce, potatoes, and carrots. Conventionally grown produce with the lowest pesticide residues include onions, avocado, frozen sweet corn, pineapples, mango, asparagus, frozen sweet peas, kiwi, bananas, cabbage, broccoli, papaya, blueberries, and cauliflower.

EIGHT

How to Raise a Healthy Eater

Parents often ask me how they can get their kids to eat well or be more active. The best advice is to start young to prevent bad habits and instill good ones. Here are recommendations for handling issues that are likely to come up at specific ages and stages of development. I suggest that you read and review them with your baby's health care provider. I tried to organize the issues according to how old your baby will be when you'll want to start thinking about them. Besides preventing bad habits, these suggestions are meant to foster your child's own ability to be an independent eater and your ability to be a responsive but not overbearing parent.

NEWBORNS

Feed your newborn on demand and allow her to self-regulate her feedings. You will be successful at this by allowing enough time to feed. Do not offer solid food. If you use a bottle, do not put anything in the bottle but the appropriate formula or expressed breast milk.

ONE TO THREE MONTHS

Your baby needs only breast milk or formula. Both have the perfect balance of nutrition. Well-meaning friends and family may give you advice about adding solids at this age, but nutritionally, your child does not need them. Avoid adding juice or solid foods unless your baby's doctor says you should.

FOUR AND FIVE MONTHS

Formula or breast milk remains the primary source of nutrition, but ask your doctor about adding solid food at this time. A baby may be developmentally able to eat, but nutritionally he does not yet require complementary foods. If you add solids, keep them simple and limited to single-ingredient foods. Serve food with a spoon, not in a bottle. Don't reduce your baby's intake of formula or breast milk just because you've introduced him to solid food. Ask your health care provider if water is needed (it usually is not). Babies do not need juice at this age, either, as it can replace the more nutrient-dense breast milk or formula.

SIX TO EIGHT MONTHS

You can start your child on solids at this time, but formula or breast milk still remains the most important part of your child's diet. Avoid combination jarred foods that are high in starch, and avoid baby desserts. Use a spoon to feed solids—never put food in a bottle, which could undermine your child's ability to self-regulate his feedings and prevent him from learning how to eat with a spoon. Learning to eat is the real reason for adding food at this age because most of your child's nutrition will still be from the milk feeding.

Do not assume that your child dislikes a food until you have offered it at least eight to fifteen times. Don't assume that just because you do not like a food, your baby won't like it, either. Now is also the time for you to take stock of your own eating habits. Your baby is already watching what you eat and how you eat. Are you sitting down to eat your own meals? Are you eating fruits and vegetables? As you start your baby on a regular feeding schedule, make sure you are in the habit, too. It is never too soon to be your child's role model.

NINE TO ELEVEN MONTHS

Introduce finger foods and appropriate table foods based on chewing ability. Encourage variety. A child offered foods that vary in textures and flavors in the first two years of life is likely to better accept new foods when she is older. Avoid foods that pose a choking risk, like hard round foods (see page 225). If you are serving juice, keep it to 6 ounces or less per day. Drinking too much juice replaces more nutritious foods. If you do serve juice, try it in a cup instead of a bottle. Do not serve soda, fruit drinks, Kool-Aid, or any sweetened beverage, even if it has claims about vitamins added.

Let your child decide how much she needs to eat. It is at about this age that some parents want to help their children eat better by controlling how much they eat. Resist that urge to control portions. Instead focus on where, what, and when your child eats. You decide where she eats (preferably sitting at a table or high chair), what she eats (include at least three different items varying in color and texture at each meal, two at snacks), and when she eats (start a loosely structured three-meal schedule and include snacks between meals). Allow her to decide how much she will eat. A regular meal and snack routine will give confidence to those of you who worry that your child will go hungry. Expect your child to eat inconsistently. It is normal for young children to eat more at one meal and less at the next. Research suggests that the too strict or overcontrolling parent may actually teach a child to doubt her ability to self-regulate, or create a preference for forbidden or controlled foods.

Habits to Put in Place in the First Year

By twelve months work toward the following routines:

- Three flexible meals with snacks in between
- Eating at a table or designated eating spot
- At least three different items at each meal, with at least one being a fruit or a vegetable; two different items for snacks, with one a fruit or vegetable

What About Sweets?

In my family, sweets did not become an issue until my girls were about fifteen months old. Prior to that, if I wanted to have a cookie, a piece of cake, or some ice cream, my children did not have enough experience with food to know they were not being offered the same food choices. When my daughter Sarah was fifteen months, my husband and I stopped for a dish of ice cream. Sarah was so curious that I gave her a taste. She loved it, and I never got my ice cream back. When dessert is served in your house, I recommend that it be made part of a meal. Your job is to serve child-size portions and protect your child from the enormous portions offered at many restaurants and ice cream shops.

Manners

Pick your battles, and be realistic and consistent. Setting limits can be tough, but your child relies on you for guidance. Manners do much more than make kids behave. Sensible manners teach sharing and cooperation.

TWELVE TO FOURTEEN MONTHS

Even at this early age children are watching and learning from what you do. The child who observes that a parent never sits to eat might interpret this to mean mealtime is not important. Start the habits of sitting down at mealtimes and acting as your baby's nutritional role model. Start reading labels; see page 56. Pay close attention to the amount of sodium in a serving of food. One-to-three-year-old children only need about 300 milligrams of sodium daily, an amount that occurs naturally in everyday food. The upper intake should not exceed 1,500 milligrams a day. One slice of pizza can have 450–1,200 milligrams of sodium, and 1 ounce of pretzels 290–560 milligrams. Avoid snacks that are actually dessert or junk food—they will cause you struggles in the future.

At twelve months you can continue to breastfeed or wean your child to whole cow's milk, but do not serve low-fat milk because children still need the calories from whole milk. Some parents prefer to continue with formula because of the nutrients it contains.

Follow these health-promoting tips:

- Offer water for thirst, not sweetened drinks like soda or fruit drinks.
- Keep offering new foods. Pair a new food with a familiar favorite.
- Look at the breads, cereal, and pastas you are offering your child. Try offering at least one to two servings of whole-grain foods per day.

FIFTEEN TO TWENTY-THREE MONTHS

This age is one of the most important times for establishing family routines. By fifteen months children can eat almost anything, but they tend to like what is familiar. Discourage the bottle and move toward a cup for milk or water. Reinforce a regular meal schedule.

Review that snack list. Be suspicious of highly advertised foods and those with nutrition claims.

Try to practice the following:

- Don't give up on variety. Offer your child a food eight to fifteen times before deciding she doesn't like it. Set a good example.
- Eat at the table and start the habit of making supper the last eating event of the day. Avoid snacks in front of the TV or computer.
- Mealtime is a time for socializing. It will be messy and chaotic, but it is a valuable teaching tool and worth the effort.
- Include dessert as part of family meals as often as you think appropriate.
- Try the "rule of one": one dessert or discretionary food per day.
- Allow your child to eat what he needs. Young children have an innate ability to eat what they need. Remember, they will eat more at one meal and less at another. Stay in the habit of offering three to five different foods at a meal and serving seconds as needed.
- Try not to use the words "good" or "bad" to describe food.
- Review the type of snacks you are offering your child.
- Is your child getting the exercise he needs? Are you active?

TWO YEARS

By age two family life will run smoother if you have a predictable meal schedule in place that includes a variety of foods. Serve appropriate portion sizes and allow for second helpings if desired. Many children can switch from whole milk to 2 percent milk now—ask your doctor.

Many parents put a TV in their child's room at a very young age. Resist the urge. Children who have a TV in their bedroom tend to be more isolated and at greater risk of being overweight because they eat more and are less active.

Try the following health-promoting tips:

- Turn the TV off at mealtimes.
- If you serve juice, offer no more than 6 ounces per day. Quench thirst with water or water flavored with a little juice or a twist of lemon or lime.
- Control the quality of meals, not the portions. Offer at least three to five different foods at meals.

THREE AND FOUR YEARS

Avoid being the food police. At mealtime, try not to critique how much or what your child is eating; save discussions about food for other times. Meals should be pleasant. If your family mealtime is a battleground, step back and take stock of what is going on. The adults in the house are responsible for setting the tone.

Avoid using food as the exclusive response to success or failure. Encourage crafts, reading a book, or taking a walk as a way to have fun, to celebrate, or to distract your child from a bad day. Get rid of the bathroom scale or move it to an out-of-the-way location. Many young children start talking about diets because they hear their mothers talking about dieting.

Keep up the following tips:

- Eat meals as a family as often as you can.
- Avoid TV at meals and limit TV to two hours per day at maximum.
- Keep to a regular meal schedule that includes all family members.
- Limit novelty foods (aka inferior foods) that are highly advertised, are highly refined, or have added sugar or other sweeteners.
- Keep offering fruits and vegetables at every meal and snack.
- Create opportunities for your children to move and be active every day.

FIVE YEARS

If you have been on a regular schedule of three meals and snacks that includes fruit and vegetable and dessert with meals, you and your family should have a very solid foundation. Now your child will be moving toward kindergarten and school lunch and snack. Most schools have improved their feeding routines quite a bit. Make sure your child gets a nutritious breakfast. Creating enough time for a morning meal will get your child off in a calm, unfrazzled manner and is worth the extra planning. Encourage a good source of calcium, and choose smart snacks. Still keep the TV out of the bedroom, limit juice, and save soda for special occasions and parties. Be active every day, and limit screen time.

PHYSICAL ACTIVITY RECOMMENDATIONS FOR ALL AGES

Human beings feel their best when their bodies are active. Engaging your child in regular forms of physical activity will prevent weight gain, prevent high blood pressure, and improve her sense of emotional well-being. A child who is active in the early years has a greater chance of being active in adulthood. The American Academy of Pediatrics recommends an hour of active play daily for children age two and older. To give your child the advantage of activity, you will have to be active yourself and plan for it with your child. Children are walking and riding bikes less today than in previous generations. We have more cars and public transportation. TV, computers, and video games replace active play. More families have two full-time working parents or one single parent, making activity or participation in classes or organized sports more difficult. Combine this with the lack of safe outdoor play areas and it is no surprise activity levels decline with age.

While your baby or toddler is young, encourage active play. When buying toys, look for push or pull toys, simple cars—these all promote movement. Encourage clapping games, tossing beanbags, or rolling a ball. Start the routine of a daily walk. Put your child in a backpack or stroller. Toddlers should get 30 minutes or more of movement daily, older kids 60 minutes or more. You can become an active family by limiting sedentary activity, taking walks on weekends, hiking, swimming, skating, or biking. Always remember kids are motivated 100 percent by fun. Joining a gym or doing sit-ups is not the way to encourage exercise among children.

The Creative Power of Boredom

Allow your child to become bored but don't allow eating as a solution. Instead turn boredom into creative play. Let your child figure out how to be creative. You can help by providing access to stimulating resources. Save big boxes—they can become forts, race cars, even homes for dolls. Keep crayons and markers on hand. Create a craft box of inexpensive supplies—feathers, ribbon, paper. Create a dress-up box from your old hand-me-downs and supplement it with fun and colorful dress-up items from the thrift shop. Have a generous supply of books, puzzles, and games on hand; swap with friends.

Protect Your Child from TV

Television has great potential for educating children, but when it comes to food and health, TV has not been part of the solution—in fact, it is part of the problem. Here are some alarming facts. Forty percent of three-month-olds watch television or videos for more than 45 minutes a day. By age two 90 percent of children are watching television for more than 90 minutes per day. Experts recommend no TV before age two. Early television viewing may interfere with a child's natural ability to interact with the real environment rather than a screen. Parents who encourage television watching may be teaching a child to be a couch potato at a very early age and increasing the risk of obesity. As your child gets older, she will be subjected to an enormous number of ads that tell her to overeat. Children between the ages of eight and twelve will see more than eight thousand food advertisements every year, and none of these will be promoting the foods they actually need, such as fruits and vegetables. Excessive television viewing limits creativity and physical activity, promotes isolation, and often allows for isolated eating. For all these reasons do not allow TV viewing before age two. When you do add TV, limit it to less than 2 hours per day, and do not put a TV in your child's bedroom.

Day Care and Babysitters

It is essential for you to share how you want your child fed when she is in the care of other people. Beyond protecting your child, your efforts to promote good nutrition can impact your larger community. Teaching everyone to sit down and eat three meals every day and to include fruits and vegetables at every meal and snack is the only way we are going to curb this obesity epidemic and diet-related disease. It is the only way we will get food companies to reinvent the prepared foods, snacks, and restaurant items they serve to us.

NINE

Effective Parenting

When my daughter Sarah was a baby, one of the smartest things I did was get involved in a mothers' group. The women in the group came from my childbirth class and a post-baby exercise class. It was the one place we could talk about babies, babies, babies, and it was a great way to learn from others. I always heard something new from these women. We often had the same concerns about parenting, but we had different solutions. This chapter is intended to be a source of ideas and information, just as I experienced twenty years ago. There is no one right way to parent, and there is often more than one answer to a problem.

ARE YOU THE PERFECT PARENT?

Yes, you are. The perfect parent is someone who cares about her child and does the best that she can with the resources she has. No one will care for and love your child as much as you do. Having a baby will challenge your patience, organization, and understanding, and for some of you parenting will make you question your abilities. This is all normal. Life with a baby in the house is not predictable. Mealtimes are interrupted, delayed, or even shortened. The scenario of calmly handing your child off to the sitter after a leisurely breakfast, with everyone in good spirits and ready to meet the day, won't always happen. The concerns that I think are important include developing pleasant mealtimes, how you speak to and about your child, teaching manners, what to do when your child says no, and how to handle a sweet tooth.

THE POWER OF THE FAMILY MEAL

The family meal provides an opportunity to connect as a family, helps children regulate their food intake, and promotes a sense of security. You might be skeptical as you sit with a baby who is flinging peas and playfully dropping the spoon. Yes, in the beginning your child will not be sharing your vision of the perfect meal, but it will be very difficult if not impossible for you to make the family meal important when your child is a teenager if you don't lay the groundwork today.

The power comes from the relationship you create. Children will obey rules and avoid high-risk behavior because of the relationship you establish, and the family table provides you with an opportunity to develop that relationship. This is very important because teens who eat with their family five times per week are less likely to smoke, drink, use drugs, or be involved in early sexual activity and more likely to have better grades. Mealtime provides the ideal opportunity to spend time together, which is important for babies and older kids. In a phone survey of teenagers asking what they worried about most, the number one concern was not having enough time with their parents. The need for parent-child connection never goes away, but busy lives—particularly work schedules and children's activities—will make getting together difficult. The family meal will always be a good way to reconnect.

As I have said before, start a family meal schedule now, but be flexible. In my house when the kids were little, the timing of breakfast varied depending on if it was a weekday or weekend, but lunch was at noon and supper at 5:00. The predictability of a schedule made life much easier in our house because the kids never had to worry about when they would eat.

CREATING A PLEASANT FAMILY MEAL

When feeding a baby, try to be organized and have everything you need ready to go. Have napkins, bowls, cups, and plates on hand and food ready to serve before you put your child in the high chair. Expect things to get messy; this is how a young child learns. Start table rules early. In my house toys were never allowed at mealtimes, at least not until my girls stopped eating.

Lots of people wonder about manners. One of the secondary benefits of eating as a family is that it requires the teaching of manners. Eating at the table calls for sharing and constraints on behavior. My rule for table manners is simple but practical. Whenever my children did something I was concerned about, I asked myself if this was behavior I could live with. For example, at the table I did not want my children taking food from a bowl with their hands. I either served them or when they were older asked them to use a spoon. If they used their hands, I took the time to correct them, and eventually they caught on. You will need to explain to children, in age-appropriate language, the type of behavior you want at the table. Children will no doubt need to be reminded of what you expect several times before they begin to internalize it.

Parents also need to set an example of good manners. When you ask your child to pass something, use respectful words such as "please" and "thank you." When you make a mistake such as spilling or breaking something, apologize—this will teach them the power of an apology. When your child does something right, compliment the positive behavior. This is often more effective than just pointing out the bad behavior. Be understanding. Your child will make mistakes, and sometimes these can be embarrassing. Just explain what can be done the next time.

Setting limits is tough, but it really helps your child to learn how to be with other human beings. Rule setting becomes an issue at fifteen to twenty-four months, and your child needs to learn what you expect. When establishing rules for behavior, you will have to develop consequences when the rules are broken. Make sure the consequences match the problem. For example, if your two-year-old runs around the house with a lollipop in her mouth, she will be breaking the "no running with food in the mouth" rule (a rule every family should have in place). Sending her to the playpen in her room for 30 minutes might not be as effective as taking away the food after you have told her to sit while eating.

Food struggles may become common now, but keep in mind that younger children are not necessarily being willful when they refuse to try a food or throw a food on the floor. In most cases they are just having fun, or they could be sick or uncomfortable. Your concerns about cleanliness and efficiency are not their concerns, and sometimes kids won't eat all you serve because they are sick or upset, the food simply does not taste good to them, or they are suspicious of how it looks.

I tried to give my kids the benefit of the doubt when they did not eat, and I tried to figure out why they were not eating. Notice if a certain behavior gets the same predictable response from you. If you offer a new food, your child does not eat much of it, and you give him macaroni and cheese instead because you know he will eat it, you might be teaching him to avoid new foods. A healthy child will get enough to eat if you keep on a predictable schedule and offer three or more foods at a meal.

THE POWER OF LANGUAGE

How you speak to and about your child will shape the relationship you create with her. I suggest that you evaluate how you speak to your child by asking if you would address an adult in the same way. You might think that you are giving away power and authority as a parent. I believe just the opposite is true—speaking to children with respect enhances parents' authority. The benefit of speaking respectfully to your children is that it sets an example and gives you the authority to ask for it back. When your child yells at you or is rude, you can say with confidence, "I do not speak to you like that, and I do not want you to speak to me in that manner, either."

Let me give you a few common meal examples. Before deciding on your toddler's menu, give her a choice about what she will be offered. Ask, "Do you want peas or carrots? Rice or noodles?" Or if you find yourself telling your child to eat all her food before she can eat dessert, try decreasing the portion size on the plate and offer an appropriately sized portion of dessert as if it is part of the meal.

Don't allow negative nicknames like "piggy" or "tubby," and don't be sarcastic. Never speak about your child as if she is not in the room. I cringe when parents talk about a child in the third person when the child is right there. Do allow your child to overhear you singing her praises. You can always find something to praise truthfully. For instance, if your child is not fond of trying new foods, instead of labeling her a "picky eater" reframe the trait into something more powerful and positive: "He hasn't found another favorite vegetable beside carrots, but he tried corn on the cob and thinks he might eat that again."

The power of language applies to the whole family. A study at the University of California at Los Angeles involved videotaping thirty-two diverse families over five years so researchers could observe how family members greeted each other coming and going. The wives stopped what they were doing to greet their spouses when they returned home only one-third of the time. Husbands greeted their wives more than half the time, but children greeted their fathers only one-third of the time. Though this is not a food issue, this study makes me want to point out the obvious: be a family that greets each other coming and going, because not doing so tells them you do not care.

TEN

Feeding Your Preschooler

Preschool-age children have a variety of unique eating issues. Growth slows down during the preschool years, and with less growth, appetite declines. This can be quite a concern to parents. Continue to get regular checkups and let your doctor reassure you about normal growth. This is also the age when children can develop food jags, when a child refuses foods that previously had been acceptable and asks for the same new food over and over. Your child may be bored with the old foods, or perhaps he is asserting his independent thinking and behavior. Do not overreact to food jags, as they are quite normal and will be only temporary. Parents should continue to select the types of food served, but you should still aim to offer a variety of food items, and include those that are tried-and-true favorites. More than ever the preschool child's appetite can vary from meal to meal and snack to snack. Keep portions small, but do offer snacks—they are very important at this age.

Peculiar trends may appear at this age, too. Many children do not like mixed foods or foods that are very hot or very cold. A sandwich that is cut the "wrong way" may be refused, and if a food item is served "out of order," such as peas before bread (or whatever else a young child thinks is the right order), it could be refused, too. When my children were this age I would not cater to every whim, but I did my best to make meals run smoothly when I could. I listened about what combinations were upsetting, and if I was cutting a sandwich, I would slice it the way they wanted it if I could. That being said, I would not throw out food just because it was not perfect, and I did not have the time to make separate meals.

As your child gets older, you will want to make sure his seat matches his size. The high chair may give way to a booster seat at this age. Cups and spoons should be part of mealtime, and dull knives may be introduced as well. Even though your child is older, I recommend you stick with unbreakable cups and plates, and continue to expect spills.

Schedules that allow adequate time for naps and a good night's sleep are still very important. A tired child will have more temper tantrums and be irritable at meals. Time snack schedules so as not to interfere with the family meal. Try to plan snacks for 1½ to 2 hours before a meal. If you get off schedule and your child is crying for something to eat close to mealtime, I recommend you serve an item that was planned as part of the meal. For example, serve sliced carrots with a little dip or a roll or slice of bread before dinner instead of with dinner, and then offer the rest of the meal as planned.

It is at this age that juice and presweetened drinks can be overconsumed and cause children to fill up on liquid calories. Keep drinks in balance. I suggest one glass of juice per day and two to three glasses of milk. Encourage water as a thirst quencher. If your child attends a day care center, the transition from day care to car to home can be very rocky if a child is tired and hungry and you are unprepared for a meal. Working parents will need to be well organized to make dinnertime run smoothly. I kept my freezer stocked with wholesome meals I'd prepared in advance, and I relied on my slow cooker.

Use the following information, adapted from the American Academy of Pediatrics' *Pediatric Nutrition Handbook,* fifth edition (2004), as a guide to balance your child's diet. If you provide the recommended number of servings from each food group on most days, your child will be eating a balanced diet. Most children will have room for more food, including dessert or snacks.

Encourage children to eat sitting down, so they can concentrate on chewing. An adult should always be supervising. Try to eliminate distractions, including loud music, toys, or games at the table. Most children will do best at learning healthy eating habits and table manners if the TV is not on. Avoid eating in the car because it will be impossible to help a child if she starts to choke; also, eating at times not associated with meals may promote overeating. Instead of using food as an activity to ease boredom, use toys, games, or music while driving and at home. Now is the time to promote active play. All young children should be active for an hour or more a day. Most just need access to a playground, a ball, or a jump rope to become active.

Feeding Two-and-Three-Year-Olds

Milk and Dairy: ½ cup milk or yogurt four to five times a day, for a total of 16–20 ounces

Meat, Fish, Poultry, or Equivalent: 1–2 ounces twice a day, for a total of 2–4 ounces

Vegetables and Fruits: four to five servings per day (a serving is 2–3 tablespoons of cooked vegetables, ½–1 small piece of fruit, 2–4 tablespoons canned fruit, or 3–4 ounces juice)

Grain Products (including whole-grain or enriched bread, cooked or dry cereal): three to four servings each day (a serving is ½–1 slice bread, ¼–½ cup cooked cereal, rice, or noodles, or ½–1 cup dry cereal)

Feeding Four-to-Six-Year-Olds

Milk and Dairy: ½–¾ cup milk or yogurt three to four times per day, for a total of 24–32 ounces

Meat, Fish, Poultry, or Equivalent: 1–2 ounces twice a day, for a total of 2–4 ounces

Vegetables and Fruits: four to five servings per day (a serving is 3–4 tablespoons of vegetables, ½–1 small piece of fruit, 4–6 tablespoons canned fruit, or 4 ounces juice)

Grain Products (including bread and cereal): three to four servings each day (a serving equals 1 slice of bread, ½ cup cooked cereal, rice, or pasta, or 1 cup dry cereal)

Fats and Oils: include some fat in the form of soft margarine, cooking oil such as canola or olive oil, nuts, or salad dressing every day.

CONTROLLING SWEET SNACKS

In 2005 the U.S. Dietary Guidelines were revised and introduced the concept of discretionary calories. Discretionary calories are the calories remaining after all the essential nutrient-dense foods have been consumed. Children ages three to six require about 1,000–1,800 calories per day (though calorie needs vary depending on activity, age, and gender). They can eat 165–195 of those calories as discretionary foods, such as ice cream, chips, candy, cookies, and so on. I think these numbers could be useful to parents trying to decide just how large a serving of brownie should be or how often chips should be allowed. The child who eats a 200-calorie package of cookies at lunch and a 200-calorie dish of ice cream at supper may be at risk of eating too much food or of being poorly nourished because the ice cream or chips are replacing more healthful foods. You can go to www.pyramid.gov to get personalized feeding advice for your child as well as yourself.

SAMPLE MEAL PLANS

Here are three sample meal plans for a four-year-old girl. The first is recommended by the American Academy of Family Physicians. The second is an example of an excessive-sugar meal plan, and the third an excessive-fat meal plan. A girl this age needs approximately 1,400 calories, 19 grams of protein, 9–25 grams of fiber, and 25–35 grams of fat. Each meal plan exceeds the protein requirement, but as you can see, fiber—an important nutrient to help with appetite control—actually drops even as total food consumption and calories climb.

Recommended Meal Plan

Breakfast	½ cup oatmeal
	4 ounces 2 percent milk
	1 orange
Snack	1 apple
	1 ounce cheese
Lunch	½ egg salad sandwich (1 boiled egg,
	1 tablespoon mayonnaise,
	1 slice wheat bread)
	4 ounces 2 percent milk
	10 baby carrots
	½ banana
Snack	½ raisin bagel
	1 tablespoon peanut butter
Supper	½ chicken breast, grilled
	½ cup peas
	½ cup cauliflower
	½ cup cooked rice
	4 ounces 2 percent milk
	¼ cantaloupe, cubed
Snack	2 slices Black Forest ham
	6 saltines
Estimated calories:	1,393
Protein:	70 grams
Fat:	43 grams
Fiber:	25 grams

Excessive Sugar

Breakfast	1 package sweetened oatmeal
	4 ounces 2 percent milk
	4 ounces orange juice
Snack	8 ounces fruit drink
	10 animal crackers
Lunch	½ egg salad sandwich
	4 ounces orange juice
	10 baby carrots

Snack	½ bagel
	1 tablespoon jam
Supper	½ chicken breast, grilled
	½ cup cooked peas
	½ cup cauliflower
	½ cup cooked rice
	4 ounces apple juice
	2 fruit-flavored strips
Snack	1 store-bought blueberry muffin
	1 tablespoon jam
Estimated calories:	1,945
Protein:	59.4 grams
Fat:	39 grams
Fiber:	21.8 grams

Excessive Fat Meal Plan

Breakfast	1 store-bought muffin with butter
	4 ounces 2 percent milk
	1 orange
Snack	1 peanut butter granola bar with chocolate coating
Lunch	½ egg salad sandwich
	½ cup chocolate pudding
	½ banana
Snack	2 ounces plain potato chips
Supper	6 chicken nuggets
	Medium order of french fries
	4 ounces 2 percent milk
	Chocolate-covered ice cream bar
Snack	2 slices Black Forest ham
	6 saltines
Estimated calories:	2,526
Protein:	66 grams
Fat:	131 grams
Fiber:	19 grams

To keep your preschooler on track, keep portions small, include vegetables with every meal, and serve fruit-based desserts most of the time when serving dessert. You will need to be proactive regarding snacks and new foods—as your child's experiences with the world outside your family grow, the outside world's influence on food choices grows, too. Don't prohibit food, but strive for good choices. When my children were this age I would let them pick out one novelty food each time we went to the store, and this was usually eaten as a dessert or part of a snack.

EVERYDAY EATING VERSUS CELEBRATORY EATING

It is perfectly okay to have fun with new foods, but distinguish between everyday eating and celebratory eating. There is room for fun food, but it can't replace superior foods too often or there will be consequences—poor food choices that can show up as excessive weight gain and diet-related health issues when your child is older.

TO GET MORE INFORMATION

The American Academy of Pediatrics has excellent information in its Parenting Corner at www.aap.org. WebMD provides information on a wide range of health issues at www.webmd.com. The Food and Nutrition Information Center offers a directory to credible, accurate resources about food and nutrition at www.nal.usda.gov/fnic. For information about parenting the older child and being successful with family meals, go to www.casa.org.

ELEVEN

Confusing Issues

When my children were babies I wanted to think that I could protect them from all illness with a good diet and a healthy environment. Obviously I could not. They got sick, and they actually needed to get sick. Routine childhood ailments are how your baby's body develops a healthy immune system and learns how to fight illness. When your child is sick, always consult a health care professional, because a serious condition could be masquerading as a routine ailment. But colds, coughs, and teething are all in your future, and comfort measures can go a long way toward making your child happier.

Health Care Professionals

Today's family can choose among a pediatrician, family doctor, nurse practitioner, and physician assistant to provide health care. I work with all of these professions and my children have received excellent care from all disciplines. The key is finding a health professional you are comfortable with.

The guidelines below are written to offer guidance on what to feed to help prevent common problems. In some cases the foods suggested may not be appropriate for infants who are under one year because they have not been exposed to the foods I suggest or they cannot chew a food as well as the older child can. Always serve foods that are appropriate in consistency and match your child's development.

WILL WHAT I FEED MY BABY NOW PREVENT DISEASE LATER?

Yes, it will. Don't let this make you feel anxious. You will see in the answers to the following health questions that the solution to preventing disease is the very same diet described in earlier chapters. We have the knowledge from years of research to make well-guided recommendations about how to prevent disease. A good diet, regular exercise, and not smoking are the cornerstones of prevention. We know that being physically active, preventing obesity, and eating well can prevent diabetes, heart disease, high blood pressure, stroke, and cancer. Good food and good habits should start early.

- Have structured but flexible meal times.
- Most days offer a fruit or vegetable with all meals and snacks.
- Replace animal fats such as butter, cream cheese, and full-fat dairy products with soft margarine, olive oil, canola oil, and low-fat dairy after age two.
- Try to make half the grain foods you serve, such as bread, cereal, or pasta, a whole-grain choice.
- Serve fish (adults should aim to eat it twice per week), poultry (without skin), beans, and nuts more often than beef or other red meats.
- After age two, switch to low-fat dairy products.
- Be active as often as possible.
- Eat dark, colorful fruits and vegetables.
- Eat as a family.

Doesn't that advice sound familiar?

DOES MY BABY NEED FIBER?

In the first year of life there is no defined fiber requirement for babies because most of their diet is in liquid form. As soon as you start adding cereal and fruit you will be adding a source of fiber. With its many health benefits, fiber will become very important, and the best sources are fruits, vegetables, and whole grains.

In the second year of life there is a little confusion about fiber recommendation. One source recommends an amount of fiber equivalent to the child's age plus 5 grams: 7 grams of fiber for a two-year-old, 10 grams for a five-year-old, and 22 grams for a seventeen-year-old. The Institute of Medicine in its Dietary Reference Intakes suggests 19 grams for one-to-three-year-olds and 25 grams for four-to-six-year-olds. You can see that the numbers are different. To help put this in perspective, consider that adults need 25–38 grams, but food surveys show that our usual intake is only about 11 grams, woefully short of what we need to be at our best health.

You can meet your toddler's fiber needs by including a fruit or vegetable at every meal and snack and including whole-grain foods at one or two meals per day. The best way to get fiber is from food because you don't have to worry if you are giving too much or too little. If your doctor recommends more fiber to correct constipation, follow those recommendations. Read about constipation on page 227.

DOES MY BABY NEED FAT?

Fat is as essential to your baby as the air he breathes. Without it he would not get the essential fatty acids and fat-soluble vitamins that keep him alive and strong. To help your child get the fat he needs, stick with formula or breast milk in the early months. As your child gets older, serve foods that are a natural source of fat, such as canola or olive oil, butter, soft margarine, cooked eggs, cooked meat or poultry or fish, nuts, yogurt, or whole milk. Fried foods are not recommended because frying adds calories but no extra nutrition, causing a child to be full but not well nourished. Read about cooking oils on page 76.

WHAT IS DHA AND HOW MUCH DHA DOES MY BABY NEED?

The fatty acid known as DHA (docosahexaenoic acid) has been mentioned earlier (see pages 26 and 82), and you will be hearing even more about it as many more products, including baby food, yogurt, and fruit drinks, put it in their ingredients list. It is a polyunsaturated fatty acid obtained from food, mainly seafood, but it may also be made in the body from an essential fatty acid called alpha-linolenic acid (ALA). DHA is now added to formula in an effort to better replicate breast milk. Breastfeeding moms who eat more fish will have more DHA in their breast milk. There is no specific guideline for DHA as there is for vitamins and minerals. Five ounces of DHA-fortified formula will contain 8–17 milligrams, and 24 ounces—an amount many one-year-olds will consume—provides 38–81 milligrams DHA. Infant foods are often fortified with 18 milligrams of DHA per serving, but fish is always a superior source. A 1-ounce portion of cooked haddock can contain 30 milligrams DHA and an ounce of salmon 200 milligrams. Some of the fat contained in canola oil, flaxseed, soybeans, and walnuts can be converted into DHA, but it is believed to be a fairly inefficient process. Fish has the additional bonus of containing EPA (eicosapentaenoic acid), another polyunsaturated fatty acid that promotes good heart health. As said earlier, finding and including sources of DHA is good for baby and the whole family.

Arachidonic acid (ARA) is a polyunsaturated fatty acid like DHA. It too is found naturally in breast milk and is added to some formulas to make it more closely resemble breast milk. It can also be derived from foods containing linoleic acid.

WHAT ABOUT OBESITY? SHOULD I BE WORRYING ABOUT IT WHEN MY CHILD IS STILL A BABY?

Don't worry about obesity, but do worry about setting a good example and laying a good foundation for eating well. To protect your child against obesity, avoid the common pitfalls that lead to weight gain: skipped or erratic meals, poor snack choices during the day, drinking a lot of high-calorie beverages, and excessive snacking after supper, while watching TV, or while on the computer. I suggest the whole family make supper the last eating event of the night; if you must eat later, make it a serving of fruit. In addition, consider these following trouble spots:

- Eat out less. A typical restaurant meal will have over 1,000 calories (and that is a lunch-size portion). That is half of an entire day's intake for most of us.
- Eat less pizza. A slice of pizza has about 400 calories. More tips for healthy pizza eating are on page 183.
- Take a walk every day.
- Eat like your baby—have three meals, include a fruit or vegetable (or both) with every meal, and serve whole-grain bread, rice, pasta, or cereal at most of your meals.
- For everyday snacks choose fruit, vegetables, or low-fat dairy between meals.
- Consume chips, fries, coffee drinks, granola bars, or soda with meals and not as snack. These foods add a tremendous amount of calories, and you will be better able to control portions when eaten as part of meal than as a snack.

CELIAC DISEASE RUNS IN MY FAMILY—WHAT SHOULD I DO TO PROTECT MY BABY?

Celiac disease, also called sprue, is a condition where the immune system identifies a protein in food called gluten as harmful. Gluten occurs in wheat, barley, and rye. When these grains are eaten, the immune system responds by causing inflammation, damaging the digestive system and causing all sorts of symptoms, from diarrhea to joint pain, skin irritations, headaches, and even delayed growth. The condition can be genetic; if it runs in your family, talk to your baby's doctor. The best time to introduce wheat, barley, or rye may be between four and six months of age, when the body can learn to handle it. Introducing gluten too soon before four months of age or delaying beyond six months might increase the risk of developing celiac disease. Simple tests can identify the problem. We now know the condition is more common than once thought, affecting almost 1 in 100 adults. The treatment is a gluten-free diet; see page 149. If your child needs a gluten-free diet, look for gluten-free grains that are enriched with B vitamins (thiamin, riboflavin, niacin, folate) and iron—read the label. For more information contact the following excellent sources: the Gluten Intolerance Group, www.gluten.net; the Celiac Disease Foundation, www.celiac.org; and the Celiac Sprue Association, www.csaceliacs.org.

SHOULD I KEEP FRUIT AND SWEETS AWAY FROM MY BABY TO PREVENT DIABETES?

Diabetes and pre-diabetes are on the rise in both children and adults, but infants and toddlers are not at great immediate risk of getting type 2 diabetes (the kind of diabetes caused by poor health habits) because the condition takes years to develop. Type 2 diabetes risk increases with age, excessive weight gain, and lack of activity.

The body makes a hormone called insulin, which helps sugar (glucose) to move from our blood into our cells, where it gives us energy. Type 2 diabetes develops when the body becomes insulin-resistant and glucose accumulates in the blood. In some cases the insulin-resistant body keeps making insulin in an attempt to lower blood sugar, a condition called hyperinsulinemia. Individuals with hyperinsulinemia, obesity, high blood pressure, and high cholesterol are at increased risk for heart disease.

If diabetes runs in your family or if you had gestational diabetes, start healthy habits today, including exercise and a good diet. Toddlers and children should enjoy active play every day, and Mom and Dad should be walking five days a week for 30 minutes a day. If you are not active now, start off slow and work up. As far as dessert and sweets go, serve child-size portions with meals and avoid snacks with a lot of sugar. The genetic predisposition to type 2 diabetes runs in families.

Type 1 diabetes usually appears in childhood and is a result of the pancreas failing to produce enough insulin. It may be triggered by environmental factors. One of them may be cow's milk protein, which has a structure similar to proteins made by the pancreas that are present before the disease develops. It has been suggested that ingesting cow's milk protein early in life, before the gut matures, could cause an immune response triggering the disease. Because the relationship between type 1 diabetes and cow's milk is not clear, the AAP has not made a recommendation on cow's milk; studies are ongoing. Breastfeed as long as you can, then follow your doctor's guidance about the type of formula to add. At age one most babies can switch to cow's milk to replace formula and use other dairy-based foods such as yogurt as part of their menu. Read about alternative calcium sources below and on page 25.

HOW MUCH DAIRY FOOD DOES MY CHILD NEED?

Children do not actually need dairy foods, but they do need calcium. Babies and infants get all the calcium they need from breast milk or formula. For older children, dairy foods are such an easy way to get calcium that they are always on the top of my list.

In the first year of life the recommended calcium intake is 210–270 milligrams per day. A child age one to three requires 500 milligrams of calcium, a four-to-eight-year-old 800 milligrams, and teenagers should get around 1,300 milligrams. The list below will show you the calcium content of dairy and nondairy foods.

Food	Calcium Content in Milligrams
Whole milk, 1 cup	291
Goat's milk, 1 cup	326
Soy milk fortified with calcium, 1 cup	300
Yogurt, 8 ounces	350
Cheese, 1 ounce	204
Dried beans, ½ cup, cooked	80
Broccoli, ½ cup, cooked	122
Tofu, ½ cup	130
Almonds, 1 ounce	73

Low-fat dairy foods carry the same amount of protein and calcium as full-fat dairy. After age two most toddlers can switch to 2 percent milk, but never start an infant on a low-fat diet.

I HAD HIGH BLOOD PRESSURE WHEN PREGNANT AND IT RUNS IN MY FAMILY—HOW CAN I PROTECT MY BABY?

High blood pressure usually carries no warning signs, which is why all adults get blood pressure screenings and all children over age three get routine blood pressure checks when they go to the doctor. High blood pressure in children is defined as a blood pressure greater than the 95th percentile for kids the same age. As you would expect, excess weight increases the risk of high blood pressure. Weight control, exercise, moderate salt intake, and a good diet are both the treatment and the prevention. Not everyone with high blood pressure is affected by sodium, but since many are, and because there is no risk to lowering sodium intake, keeping sodium at the Dietary Reference Intake (DRI) level of less than 1 gram for toddlers is wise.

EVERYBODY TALKS ABOUT LOWERING CHOLESTEROL—SHOULD I KEEP EGGS AWAY FROM MY BABY?

Serve your child eggs, because they are a superb protein source. Just hold the bacon and sausage. Adults with high levels of total and LDL ("bad") cholesterol increase their risk of coronary artery disease and heart attacks. One-third of adults who have a heart attack have total cholesterol above 250. Children with high cholesterol levels are likely to become adults with high cholesterol levels, increasing their risk of early heart disease.

Fruit and vegetables are plant foods, so they carry no cholesterol. They do provide fiber, which can lower blood cholesterol levels. Foods made from whole grains can lower cholesterol, too. Limit foods high in saturated fat. Saturated fat is the type of fat found in most animal foods, and it raises cholesterol. Plant-based foods rich in polyunsaturated fats and monounsaturated fats, such as olives, soft margarine, canola oil, olive oil, and nuts, do not raise cholesterol.

I HAVE HEARD THERE IS A SUBSTANCE IN WHOLE GRAINS AND SOY PRODUCTS THAT ACTS AS AN ANTI-NUTRIENT—IS THAT TRUE?

Phytic acid is a natural plant chemical found in the hulls of seeds, nuts, and grains. It can block the absorption of calcium, iron, magnesium, and zinc, which could pose obvious nutrition problems, but this same property may be the reason it seems to reduce the risk of some forms of cancer. An article in the *American Journal of Clinical Nutrition* notes that eating foods high in phytic acid as part of an adequate diet did not cause nutrient deficiencies. Since seeds, nuts, and whole grains are nutrient-dense foods credited with preventing disease, they should be part of the family menu.

IS THERE A DIET TO PREVENT ASTHMA?

Asthma is a chronic lung condition characterized by symptoms of wheezing, shortness of breath, difficulty breathing, and coughing. The prevalence of asthma among American children has increased from 3.6 percent in 1980 to 5.8 percent in 2003. There is no one clinical measurement that identifies asthma with certainty. A doctor makes the diagnosis based on medical history, a physical examination, and the exclusion of other diagnoses that might explain the symptoms. Secondhand smoke has consistently been shown to impact the diagnosis of asthma. Allergies to dust mites and pet dander may also contribute to asthma symptoms. Some research suggests exposing your child early on to animals may decrease the risk of asthma; this is not rock solid, but if you are thinking of having a family pet, maybe getting one sooner rather than later is a good idea. Exposure to air pollution can exacerbate asthma symptoms and increase rates of hospitalization, but whether asthma is caused by pollution or aggravated by it is not clear. Pollution from automobiles may have more of an impact than pollution from industry such as coal emissions.

The connection between diet and asthma is not clear or simple. There is a parallel trend in both obesity and asthma that is most consistent among adolescent girls; researchers think being overweight precedes the asthma, not that asthma leads to inactivity and thus to overweight. While at one time it was thought that avoiding cow's milk and eggs during pregnancy reduced the child's risk of asthma, we now know that this is not true. Eating foods rich in omega-3 fatty acids such as fish and eating yogurt fortified with lactobacilli (probiotics) has been shown to reduce eczema and might be associated with less asthma. Authorities recommend avoiding secondhand smoke as a prevention strategy.

DO I NEED TO BRUSH MY BABY'S TEETH?

Over 95 percent of Americans have cavities, and as soon as your child's first tooth erupts, around four to six months, she can get them, too. Cavities occur when decay-causing bacteria collect in the sticky substance called plaque. When your child eats a sweet or starchy food the bacteria release an acid that can cause a cavity. The longer a tooth is in contact with that acid, the greater the chance a cavity can form. That is why brushing to remove the plaque needs to become an early habit.

To avoid cavities:

- Clean your child's teeth with gauze or an infant toothbrush twice a day once teeth emerge.
- Give only water before naptime or bedtime. Milk, formula, juice, or soda all contain carbohydrate, the nutrient bacteria thrive on. Liquids can be a particular problem because they bathe the whole tooth and even get in between teeth.
- When your child eats sticky foods such as dried fruit, fruit leather, or gummy bears, brush her teeth or at the very least have her rinse.
- Avoid sugary snacks in favor of snacks with some protein, such as cheese, nuts, or a hard-boiled egg.
- Foods that require lots of chewing, such as peppers, cucumbers, celery, and carrots, are great choices.
- Popcorn, plain crackers, and rice cakes are less likely to cause cavities than cookies, candy, or granola bars.

It is not possible to feed your child a sugar-free diet. Sugars occur naturally in milk, bread, and fruit. It is good to reduce added sugars, but even with the best of diets children still have to brush.

HOW CAN I AVOID THE RISK OF CHOKING?

The same practices that minimize the risk of choking can also promote good eating. Sitting in one location to eat reduces the risk of choking because it improves concentration on chewing and swallowing; it also eliminates distractions that can lead to a habit of mindless eating.

Hard round foods must be controlled because they can lodge in the throat, acting like a dangerous plug. Such foods include nuts, raw carrots, popcorn, round candy, hot dogs, grapes, and string cheese. Before serving any of these items slice them longitudinally into slivers, not horizontally into coins. You don't want to always chop everything up—the older child needs to learn how to chew—but preventing choking by slicing will not slow development. Your child should be given foods that match her ability to feed herself. When a child is eating, an adult should always be present and within reach. Also, be aware that rub-on teething medications can interfere with chewing and swallowing because they can cause numbness of the muscles in the throat.

DO DAIRY PRODUCTS CAUSE COLIC?

In a healthy infant, colic is defined as inconsolable crying for no apparent reason more than three hours per day for more than three days per week and for more than three weeks. Most doctors believe the problem is the result of an immature digestive tract. The good news is that the condition does no harm and your baby will outgrow it, usually around three months of age. You, on the other hand, are likely to find the crying to be a tremendous source of stress. There is no simple or guaranteed solution, but do discuss the problem with your doctor, just to be sure there is no underlying cause for the crying.

Many parents will want to change formulas, hoping that changing from a cow's-milk-based formula to a soy-based one might give relief, but this is not recommended by the AAP because it has not been found to be consistently effective and infants may develop an allergy to soy. The most common medicine prescribed is an over-the-counter product called simethicone (Mylicon), used to decrease intestinal gas. However, a trial reported in the journal *Pediatrics* concluded that the drug was no more effective than a placebo. Many parents swear by herbal tea as a colic treatment, but since herbal products may not be well standardized, the dosage may be an issue. Also, be aware that tea that contains no calories, protein, or other nutrients may displace formula or breast milk. What is called "gripe water" contains a variety of herbs and oils. These are not endorsed products, but if you try one, choose a product without alcohol or sugar and manufactured in the United States, and make sure it does not interfere with breastfeeding or formula feeding.

Saying there is no cure for colic is not the same as saying there is nothing to be done. Car rides, white noise, and swaddling are time-honored treatments, and since they do no harm and some parents report them to be effective, why not try the following?

- Hold your baby close. Place him in a backpack while you do chores. Some parents swear by the "football hold"—support the baby on your forearm, stomach down, baby's head in your hand, and legs dangling.
- Rock your child in a rocker.
- Do not stop breastfeeding just because your baby is colicky. Some breastfeeding mothers find eating cruciferous vegetables (broccoli, Brussels sprouts, cabbage, cauliflower, rutabaga, and turnips), onions, chocolate, and cow's milk are associated with colic. Limiting these foods is not unreasonable. Just choose other vegetables and replace cow's milk with another good calcium source.
- Try to keep your infant on a flexible but established feeding schedule. If you are bottle-feeding, ask your doctor about the size of the hole in the nipple. If the hole is the wrong size, your baby might be swallowing too much air.
- Babies who burp or pass gas seem to feel better and cry less.
- Avoid secondhand smoke.
- Keep calm. One of my most stressful periods as a new parent was when my older daughter had colic. The crying and inability to console her were terribly distressing, and no activity could distract me from my anxieties. Watching the evening

news with headphones and my crying baby in my arms was the best I could do.

MY TWELVE-MONTH-OLD WON'T EAT ANYTHING BUT WHITE FOOD— BREAD, NOODLES, AND CHEESE

The first question would be whether the child has a developmental issue such as sensory or swallowing problems. If the child is healthy and growing well, then he probably has simply become familiar with these foods and likes them best. Next time you feed your child, include colored foods on the plate—grated carrots, a sliced grape, whatever you are eating. Don't make a fuss about it, but do make it part of everyday eating. Eventually the food will start to look familiar and he will try it.

I THINK MY BABY IS CONSTIPATED— WHAT SHOULD I DO?

You are in good company if you worry about your child's bowel movements. Constipation is responsible for 3–5 percent of children's visits to doctors each year. As children get older, expect the frequency of bowel movements to decline. In infants the mean daily number of BMs is 2.2 and in one-to-three-year-olds the mean is 1.4. Breast-fed babies tend to have slightly more bowel movements than formula-fed infants. But just because your child has less frequent BMs does not mean he is actually constipated. The frequency of BMs varies tremendously. It is the presence of hard dry stools that cause discomfort that is the problem. Remember that it is normal for a baby to make a face and get red when having a BM, so don't be alarmed.

Most cases of constipation are considered "functional," meaning there is not an underlying medical problem. Fear of having a bowel movement is probably the most common reason children retain feces. This fear may develop when a child passes a large or hard stool that causes pain or a small tear in the anus. Constipation is very rarely an attempt by a child to be oppositional. Always discuss the problem with your pediatrician to allay your fears.

Your pediatrician can treat constipation with disimpaction, oral medication, suppositories, or enemas. The goal is to maintain soft bowel movements, aiming for regularity so that the cycle of constipation does not repeat itself. It might surprise you to learn that constipation can be hard to treat—30 to 50 percent of children who have been treated for constipation have a recurrence of the problem later on. If your doctor advises more fiber, ask for specific guidance on type and amount. Psyllium seed husks and bran fiber can be effective but must be taken with a lot of water. I prefer fruit and cooked whole grains because they combine both fiber and water naturally.

Food	Fiber (in grams)
½ cup applesauce	2
1 medium avocado	8–16
½ cup blueberries	2
½ cup cooked brown rice	2

When you move into the toilet-training years, be patient with your child. Constipation can be a problem at this stage because a busy child may ignore the urge to defecate. When the urge to defecate is ignored, it goes away, and if this is done too often constipation can result. Keep your toilet-trained child on a schedule. By that I mean just make sure he has the time and opportunity to use the toilet—it doesn't matter if he goes every time, just that he can if he needs to. And for those of you who worry your child will never be toilet-trained—relax, I promise they all learn how to do it. Some are just faster than others.

- Once your child is on solid foods serve a fruit or vegetable with meals and snacks and serve whole-grain foods with at least one meal per day.

- Make sure your child gets enough fluid. Fruit, vegetables, and cooked grains have the added benefit of providing fiber plus a natural source of fluid.
- If you mix your own formula, make sure it is not overconcentrated.
- Serve natural laxatives. Try the recipe for Yogurt with Prune Sauce on page 126, or any cooked fruit recipe.
- Constipation may be related to milk intolerance in some children. Ask your doctor about trying a cow's-milk-free menu for a short time to see if it helps. Read about eliminating cow's milk on page 24.
- Physical activity improves digestion and defecation, so instill good habits early.
- Do not give your child a laxative without the doctor's guidance.

Encopresis is the involuntary release of feces into undergarments. Thirty-five percent of girls and 55 percent of boys who are constipated may also experience this problem. Encopresis is an involuntary action that is probably as upsetting to a five-year-child as it is to a parent.

WHAT SHOULD I GIVE MY BABY WHEN HE HAS DIARRHEA?

Diarrhea, or frequent watery bowel movements, can be caused by food or beverages, viruses, bacteria, even teething. It can be serious if it causes dehydration (the loss of too much fluid from the body). Most cases of diarrhea do not lead to dehydration, but it is important to be aware of the signs and prevent it by offering fluids. The signs of dehydration can include no wet diapers or no urinating, dark urine, and no tears when crying. Infants under eighteen months can have a sunken soft spot on their head. Of course poor appetite, irritability, and weight loss can occur as well.

Most babies should stay on their usual breast milk or formula feedings when ill. In some cases the doctor might advise diluting formula or even trying lactose-free formula or lactose-free milk. If formula is diluted, it should be for only a short period, because calories will be reduced.

To replace fluids in a child over two, offer clear liquids, including water, broth, ginger ale, white grape juice, herbal tea, Jell-O (not sugar-free), water ice, or Popsicles. Avoid foods or beverages with sorbitol (prune, pear, cherry, and apple juice are natural sources), and avoid drinks with caffeine, including colas or regular teas because the caffeine acts as a mild diuretic. Oral rehydraton solution (ORS) such as Pedialyte provides a balanced mix of sodium, potassium, and sugar. For infants, make sure you get guidance on the use of these products, as they are very low in calories. Follow your doctor's advice, but return to a regular diet within 12 to 24 hours. Breast-fed infants can continue to nurse while on ORS, and formula-fed babies drinking ORS instead of formula on the advice of the doctor should do so for no more than 12 to 24 hours. If diarrhea is severe and your child has trouble keeping anything down, try offering liquids in very small amounts, as little as 1 teaspoonful at a time. Older children may like ice chips to chew on.

Continue to offer your child his usual diet, including formula or breast milk if an infant is not fully weaned. Good foods to offer can include bland, soft foods such as rice, pasta, or potatoes and lean protein such as cooked egg or chicken. Avoid foods with a high sugar content or a high fat content

The BRATT (bananas, rice, applesauce, tea, toast) diet is no longer recommended to treat diarrhea because it is not well balanced and it is low in calories, but you can still offer your child any of these foods along with his regular diet.

Chronic Nonspecific Diarrhea

If your child has sloppy stools that consist of three or more mucous bowel movements daily, she may have an increasingly common condition called chronic nonspecific diarrhea. It occurs in children six months to three years old and spontaneously self-corrects after age three. It is common for it to occur among siblings. Fortunately, it appears not to impact growth or health. Do call it to your doctor's attention so that the possibility of an underlying health problem can be ruled out, but if your child is given this diagnosis, take comfort in the fact that it is common and will be outgrown. There are a few dietary precautions that might limit the number of bowel movements. Limit total juice consumption to 4 to 8 ounces per day. Avoid prune, pear, cherry, or apple juice because of their higher content of sorbitol, a naturally occurring sugar alcohol linked to diarrhea. Eliminate milk only if you have identified it as increasing diarrhea. Offer a regular diet including all food groups needed for your child's age.

WHAT SHOULD I FEED MY CHILD WHEN SHE HAS A FEVER?

Fevers are unavoidable, so be prepared for them. Have an infant thermometer in the house and bring it with you when you travel. The first thing your child's doctor will ask when you call with the complaint of a fever is exactly how high it is. You cannot determine this by touch; you must use a thermometer. At your early baby checkups ask your doctor what over-the-counter medicines are recommended to treat fever. Having these in the house means you will not have to take your sick infant to the drugstore to get it. Most of the time fever accompanies a routine ailment that can be managed at home, but that is not always the case. Sometimes fever is the first sign of a serious illness. In very young children less than two months of age a fever above 100.4°F requires a call to the doctor. In an older child that same fever may not be such a cause for alarm, but ask your baby's doctor for guidance.

Older children with fever can benefit from clear soothing liquids such as ginger ale. Most infants will be advised to stick with formula or breast milk. Oral rehydration solution may be advised, but follow the doctor's advice. If in addition to the fever your child cannot keep fluids down because of vomiting, she may be at risk of dehydration, and oral rehydration solution may be needed.

GASTROESOPHAGEAL REFLUX

Gastroesophageal reflux (GER), the regurgitation or "spitting up" of stomach contents, is common in infants. It usually begins between one and four months, and it resolves by six to twelve months. In fact, it is so common that 40 to 65 percent of healthy infants are likely to have it in the early months of their life, but by one year that number drops to 1 percent. Babies with GER maintain normal weight gain and have no breathing difficulties, and the reflux does not irritate the esophagus (esophagitis). Pediatricians are likely to suggest thickening the formula with cereal and feeding the baby in an upright position to allow gravity to help prevent symptoms. Smaller frequent feedings are often advised. Some physicians will recommend a short trial of casein hydrolysate formula if a cow's milk allergy is suspected in GER.

Though GER occurs in the majority of babies, about one in three hundred infants will have similar reflux symptoms associated with poor weight gain, esophagitis, and respiratory symptoms (cough and wheezing). This is called gastroesophageal reflux disease (GERD). GERD is distinguished from GER by these secondary symptoms. The poor growth probably occurs because eating is associated with regurgitation, which can be painful, and if eating is associated with discomfort, the baby will learn not to eat in order to avoid the pain. GERD is probably caused by a relaxed esophageal sphincter, which normally keeps stomach contents from washing back up into the esophagus. When GERD is suspected, upper GI examination may be considered. This can involve examining the esophagus with a probe (endoscopy) or a biopsy. In some cases a trial of medication will be done, and if it gives relief it will be continued.

IRON-DEFICIENCY ANEMIA

Healthy babies are born with enough stored iron to meet their need for growth up until about four to six-plus months of age. Breast milk carries a highly absorbable form of iron, and formula has iron added to it, but starting around four months all infants can benefit from a food source. For this reason first foods should contain a source of iron. Infant cereal fortified with iron is the most popular first food.

Iron deficiency anemia (a more serious condition) affects about 3 percent of children age one to three years. An iron deficiency can impact motor development, behavior, and cognitive ability. For children at risk for deficiency, supplements may be advised, along with foods rich in iron.

Two forms of iron exist in food: heme iron, which is found in meat, and non-heme iron, found in plant foods. Heme iron is well absorbed, while non-heme iron absorption can be affected by other food components. Calcium, fiber, and polyphenols and tannins (found in tea, coffee, and wine) inhibit absorption, while vitamin C improves it, as does even a small amount of meat. The DRI for healthy adults is 8 milligrams per day, but vegetarian adults are advised to ingest 16 milligrams per day, because much of their iron will be in the form of non-heme iron.

To prevent iron deficiency and iron deficiency anemia:

- Breastfeed as long as possible.
- Offer a good food source of iron starting at four to six months.
- Formula-fed infants should be given only iron-fortified formula.
- Avoid cow's milk in the first twelve months of life, and for older children make sure milk does not replace iron-rich foods.
- Ensure a good intake of vitamin C to promote the absorption of non-heme iron. Oranges, grapefruit, cantaloupe, strawberries, broccoli, green beans, and peppers are good sources of vitamin C.

LACTOSE INTOLERANCE

Lactose, or milk sugar, is the primary carbohydrate in all mammalian milks. Most babies produce an enzyme called lactase that helps digest lactose. Only very rarely are infants born with the inability to digest lactose. (Preterm infants may not digest lactose as well as other forms of sugar. Read about feeding the preterm infant on page 20). However, with age and sometimes with illness, problems tolerating lactose can develop. Symptoms of lactose intolerance can include flatulence, bloating, abdominal pain, nausea, and vomiting. These symptoms occur when lactose goes undigested from the small intestine into the large intestine, where it is acted on by normal intestinal bacteria. Asians, African Americans, and Hispanics are more likely to have a problem with lactose intolerance than whites. A decline in lactase production usually begins between three and seven years. However, most people can tolerate lactose when consumed in small portions, ½ to 1 cup at a time. Yogurt and cheeses pose less of a problem because the friendly bacteria used to culture them break down some of the lactose.

Infants can have a problem with lactose when they have stomach ailments that result in diarrhea. Diarrhea irritates the intestine, stripping it of lactase and making it difficult to digest lactose. Infants who have this trouble may be advised to avoid lactose for a while. This is done by switching to a lactose-free formula for 1–2 weeks, until the problem clears.

For children who cannot tolerate lactose, nondairy sources of calcium can include fortified soy milk, nuts, leafy greens, fortified cereal, even molasses and maple syrup. Read about calcium on page 25.

STOMACHACHE

A stomachache can be caused by illness, overeating, constipation, and even stress. Lack of fiber, lack of fluids, too much of one food, or irregular meals can all be factors. Inform your doctor if your child's stomachache is accompanied by fever, vomiting, diarrhea, or injury. When a medical reason has been ruled out, look to diet.

- Get meals and snacks on a regular schedule.
- Try more whole grains.
- For adequate fiber, offer a fruit or vegetable at every meal or snack.
- Offer the right fluids. Avoid those with high sugar content,

such as fruit juice, fruit drinks, and particularly milk shakes. Instead, try plain water or herb tea sweetened with a small amount of honey (for children over one year of age)

· Sit down at meals, and encourage adequate chewing and sufficient time for digestion.

If stress is an issue, don't ignore it—a tummyache caused by anxiety or nerves is just as real as one caused by illness. Movement is a great stress reliever. Dance to a fun song, take a walk, practice deep breathing, watch a funny movie, and reassure your child.

VOMITING

Vomiting can be caused by illnesses (whether from viruses or from bacteria), by foods that are hard to handle because they are too sweet, or by foods that have been contaminated. In many ways vomiting is a natural protective defense—the body tries to expel a problematic food—but it can be serious if it is frequent and leads to dehydration. To prevent dehydration, your child needs fluids.

Your doctor may recommend oral rehydration solution. Breast-fed and formula-fed babies are usually given their regular feeding along with ORS.

If vomiting persists, try giving fluids in small amounts. An infant who is hungry or thirsty may consume too much too fast when given a bottle, and vomiting may occur again. A teaspoon of fluid given every few minutes may stay down better, but you will have to get the total volume recommended into your baby. Make sure you call your baby's doctor if your baby is vomiting and younger than six months, or if vomiting persists, if it occurs with great force, or if your child could have swallowed something that was poisonous.

NITRATE POISONING

Nitrate poisoning can result in a serious condition called methemoglobinemia. Most cases in the United States have occurred when water from a nitrate-contaminated well has been used to prepare infant formula. More than fifteen million families rely on well water that is not subject to standards or testing, and many of these wells may not meet the federal drinking water standard for nitrate. Any family consuming water from a private well should have the water tested for nitrate.

Food occasionally has been a source of nitrate poisoning though it does not pose nearly the risk well water does. In the United States only one case of food-related nitrate poisoning (from carrot juice) has been reported. Nitrates occur naturally in some plants, including green beans, carrots, squash, spinach, and beets. Commercially prepared infant vegetables are monitored for nitrate level and are safe for babies. Home preparation of any of these foods should be avoided until your baby is at least three months of age (though, as I have noted, there is no nutritional need to add any solid foods before four months).

After three months the risk of nitrate poisoning diminishes as the baby's digestive tract matures. In older children and adults, nitrate poisoning is no longer a concern, as the substance can be safely absorbed and excreted by the body.

References

The feeding recommendations are adapted from the following general pediatric nutrition references:

American Academy of Pediatrics, Committee on Nutrition. *Pediatric Nutrition Handbook,* 5th ed. Elk Grove Village, IL: American Academy of Pediatrics, 2004.

American Dietetic Association. *Manual of Clinical Dietetics,* 6th ed. Chicago: American Dietetic Association, 2000.

Krause's Food, Nutrition, and Diet Therapy, Mahan, L. K., and S. Escott-Stump, eds., 11th ed. New York: Elsevier, 2004.

These books provided insight and inspiration and are recommended reading for anyone interested in the interrelation of food, obesity, and parenting:

Critser, Greg. *Fat Land: How Americans Became the Fattest People in the World.* Boston: Houghton Mifflin, 2003.

Nestle, Marion. *What to Eat.* New York: North Point Press, 2006.

Satter, Ellyn. *Your Child's Weight: Helping Without Harming, Birth Through Adolescence.* Madison, WI: Kelcy Press, 2005.

Shell, Ellen Ruppel. *The Hungry Gene: The Science of Fat and the Future of Thin.* New York: Atlantic Monthly Press, 2002.

INTRODUCTION

Bazzano, L. The High Cost of Not Consuming Fruits and Vegetables. *Journal of the American Dietetic Association* 106, 9 (2006): 1364–1379.

Brownell, K. *Food Fight: The Inside Story of the Food Industry, America's Obesity Crisis, and What We Can Do About It.* New York: McGraw-Hill, 2003.

CHAPTER 1: THIS IS NOT YOUR MOTHER'S KITCHEN

Devaney, B., L. Kalb, R. Briefel, et al. Feeding Infants and Toddlers Study: Overview of the Study Design. *Journal of the American Dietetic Association* 104, 1 (2004): S8–S13.

Dwyer, J. T., C. W. Suitor, and K. Hendricks. FITS: Insights and Lessons Learned. *Journal of the American Dietetic Association* 104, 1 (2004): S5–S7.

Food Illusions: Why We Eat More than We Think. *Nutrition Action Healthletter* 11, 2 (2004): 1, 3–6.

Fox, M. K., S. Pac, B. Devaney, et al. Feeding Infants and Toddlers Study: What Foods Are Toddlers Eating? *Journal of the American Dietetic Association* 104, 1 (2004): S22–S30.

Liebman, B. Defensive Eating: Staying Lean in a Fattening World. *Nutrition Action Healthletter* 8, 10 (2001): 1, 3–8.

Nestle, Marion. *What to Eat.* New York: North Point Press, 2006.

Wright, J. D., C. Y. Wang, J. Kennedy-Stephenson, et al. Dietary Intake of Ten Key Nutrients for Public Health, United States: 1999–2000. Advance Data from Vital and Health Statistics, no. 334. Hyattsville, MD: National Center for Health Statistics, 2003.

CHAPTER 2: THE EASY YEAR

American Heart Association, S. S. Gidding, B. A. Dennison, et al. Dietary Recommendations for Children and Adolescents: A Guide for Practitioners. *Pediatrics* 117 (2006): 544–559. Available at www.pediatrics.org/cgi/content/full/117/2/544.

Bodnar, L. M. The High Prevalence of Vitamin D Insufficiency in Black and White Pregnant Women Residing in Northern United States and Their Neonates. *Journal of Nutrition* 137, 2 (2007): 305–306.

Breen, F. M. Heritability of Food Preferences in Young Children. *Physiology and Behavior* 88, 4–5 (2006): 443–447.

Butte, N., K. Cobb, J. Dwyer, et al. The Start Healthy Feeding Guidelines for Infants and Toddlers. *Journal of the American Dietetic Association* 104, 3 (2004): 442–454.

Mangels, A. R., and V. Messina. Considerations in Planning Vegan Diets: Infants. *Journal of the American Dietetic Association* 101, 6 (2001): 670–677.

Puntis, J. W. L. Nutritional Support in the Premature Newborn. *Postgraduate Medical Journal* 82, 965 (2006): 192–198.

Saenz, R. B. Primary Care of Infants and Young Children with Down Syndrome. *American Family Physician* 59, 2 (1999). Available at www.aafp.org/afp/990115ap/381.html.

CHAPTER 3: FEEDING YOUR TODDLER

Allen, R. E., and A. L. Myers. Nutrition in Toddlers. *American Family Physician* 74, 9 (2006): 1527–1532.

Breen, F. M., R. Plomin, and J. Wardle. Heritability of Food Preferences in Young Children. *Journal of Physiology and Behavior* 88, 4–5 (2006): 443–447.

Carruth, B. R., P. J. Ziegler, A. Gordon, et al. Developmental Milestones and Self-Feeding Behaviours in Infants and Toddlers. *Journal of the American Dietetic Association* 104, 1 (2004): S51–S56.

———. Prevalence of Picky Eaters Among Infants and Toddlers and Their Caregivers' Decisions About Offering a New Food. *Journal of the American Dietetic Association* 104, 1 (2004): S57–S64.

Cooke, L. J. Genetic and Environmental Influences on Children's Food Neophobia. *American Journal of Clinical Nutrition* 86, 2 (2007): 428–433.

Savage, J. S., J. O. Fisher, and L. L. Birch. Parental Influence on Eating Behavior: Conception to Adolescence. *Journal of Law, Medicine and Ethics* 35, 1 (2007): 22–34.

Skinner, J. D., P. Ziegler, S. Pac, et al. Meal and Snack Patterns of Infants and Toddlers. *Journal of the American Dietetic Association* 104, 1 (2004): S65–S70.

CHAPTER 4: SUPERIOR FOODS

Much of the buying and cooking information for the foods is from the USDA Agricultural Marketing Service, www.ams.usda.gov; search on "How to Buy Fruits and Vegetables."

CHAPTER 7: HOW TO SHOP

"Certified Humane" Food Label Unveiled. Press release, May 22, 2003. Available at www.hsus.org/press_and_publications/press_releases/certified_humane_food_label_unveiled.html.

Deciphering Organic Labeling. Available at www.eatright.org/cps/rde/xchg/ada/hs.xsl/home_11028_ENU_Print.htm.

Economic Policy Institute Basic Family Budget Calculator. Available at www.epinet.org.

Environmental Working Group. Best Produce. Available at www.foodnews.org/.

———. Mercury in Seafood. Available at www.exg.org/news/story.php?print-version +1&id+5551.

Extension Toxicology Network. Food Quality Protection Act (FQPA). Available at http://extoxnet.orst.edu/faqs/.

McCann, D. Food Additives and Hyperactive Behaviour in Three-Year-Old and Eight/Nine-Year-Old Children in the Community: A Randomized, Double-Blinded, Placebo-Controlled Trial. *Lancet* 3; 370, 9598 (2007): 1560–1567.

Mendoza, M. Nutrition Class Not Curbing Junk-Food Craving. *Boston Globe,*

July 5, 2007, www.boston.com/yourlife/health/children/articles/2007/07/05/nutrition_class (accessed January 20, 2008).

Nestle, Marion. *What to Eat.* New York: North Point Press, 2006.

Organic Food—Better for Baby? *Consumer Reports.* www.consumerreports.org/cro/health-fitness/exercise-wellness/consumer-reports-why-organic-baby-food-is-safer-106/overview/index.htm.

Organic Trade Association. Nutritional Considerations. Available at www.ota.com/organic/benefits/nutrition.html.

USDA. Organic Food Standards and Labels: The Facts. Available at www.ams.usda.gov/nop/Consumers/brochure.html.

CHAPTER 8: HOW TO RAISE A HEALTHY EATER

Agras, S. W. Influence of Early Feeding Style on Adiposity at 6 Years of Age. *Journal of Pediatrics* 116, 5 (1990): 805–809.

American Academy of Pediatrics, Committee on Nutrition. *Pediatric Handbook,* 5th ed. Elk Grove Village, IL: American Academy of Pediatrics, 2003–2004.

——. Policy Statement: Prevention of Pediatric Overweight and Obesity. *Pediatrics* 112, 2 (2003): 424–430.

American Academy of Pediatrics, Committee on Public Education. Children, Adolescents, and Television. *Pediatrics* 107, 2 (2001): 423–426.

Birch, L. Development of Eating Behaviors Among Children and Adolescents. *Pediatrics* 101, 3, pt. 2 (1998): 539–549.

Bowman, S. A., S. L. Gortmaker, C. A. Ebbeling, et al. Effects of Fast-Food Consumption on Energy Intake and Diet Quality in a National Household Survey. *Pediatrics* 113, 1 (2004): 112–118.

Butte, N., K. Cobb, J. Dwyer, et al. The Start Healthy Feeding Guidelines for Infants and Toddlers. *Journal of the American Dietetic Association* 104, 3 (2004): 442–454.

Columbus Children's Hospital. Childhood Obesity Expert Recommends Simple Interventions. Oct. 21, 2002. Available at http://www.newswise.com/articles/2002/10/obesity.coh.html.

Meltz, B. Heavy TV Viewing Under 2 Is Found. *Boston Globe,* May 27, 2007.

Mendoza, M. Nutrition Class Not Curbing Junk-Food Craving. *Boston Globe,* July 5, 2007, www.boston.com/yourlife/health/children/articles/2007/07/05/nutrition_class (accessed January 20, 2008).

Rolls, B. J., D. Engell, and L. Birch. Serving Portion Size Influences 5-Year-Old but Not 3-Year-Old Children's Food Intakes. *Journal of the American Dietetic Association* 100, 2 (2000): 232–234.

Satter, E. M. Internal Regulation and the Evolution of Normal Growth as the Basis for Prevention of Obesity in Children. *Journal of the American Dietetic Association* 96, 9 (1996): 860–864.

Schreiber, G. B. Weight Modification Efforts Reported by Black and White Preadolescent Girls: National Heart, Lung, and Blood Institute Growth and Health Study. *Pediatrics* 98, 1 (1996): 63–70.

Surgeon General of the United States. The Surgeon General's Call to Action to Prevent and Decrease Overweight and Obesity. Rockville, MD: US DHHS Public Health Service, Office of the Surgeon General, 2001, www.surgeongeneral .gov/library.

Williams, C. L., L. L. Hayman, S. R. Daniels, et al. American Heart Association Scientific Statement: Cardiovascular Health in Childhood. *Circulation* 106, 1 (2002): 143–60.

CHAPTER 9: EFFECTIVE PARENTING

Fulkerson, J. A., D. Neumark-Sztainer, and M. Story. Adolescent and Parent Views of Family Meals. *Journal of the American Dietetic Association* 106, 4 (2006): 525–533.

Gillman, M. W., S. L. Rifas-Shiman, A. L. Frazier, et al. Family Dinner and Quality Among Older Children and Adolescents. *Archives of Family Medicine* 9, 3 (2000): 235–240.

National Center on Addiction and Substance Abuse at Columbia University (CASA). Family Meals. Available at www.casafamilyday.org.

Patton, S. R., L. M. Dolan, and S. W. Powers. Relationships Between Use of Television During Meals and Children's Food Consumption Patterns. *Pediatrics* 107, 1 (2001): E7.

CHAPTER 10: FEEDING YOUR PRESCHOOLER

Allen, R. E., and A. L. Myers. Nutrition in Toddlers. *American Family Physician* 74, 9 (2006): 1527–1532.

CHAPTER 11: CONFUSING ISSUES

American Academy of Family Physicians. Managing Fever Without Source in Infants and Children. Available at www.aafp.org/afp/20010601/tips/10.html.

———. Vomiting and Diarrhea in Children. Available at www.aafp.org/ afp/ 20010215/775ph.html.

American Heart Association. Scientific Statement: Cardiovascular Health in Childhood. *Circulation* 106 (2002): 143–160. Available at http://circ.ahajournals .org/cgi/content/full/106/1/143.

Biggs, W. S., and W. H. Dery. Evaluation and Treatment of Constipation in Infants and Children. *American Family Physician* 73 (2006): 469–477, 479–480, 481–482.

Eder, W., M. J. Ege, and E. V. von Mutius. The Asthma Epidemic. *New England Journal of Medicine* 355 (2006): 2226–2235.

Greer, F. R., and M. Shannon. Infant Methemoglobinemia: The Role of Dietary Nitrate in Food and Water. *Pediatrics* 116, 3 (2005): 784–786.

Hunt, J. R. Bioavailability of Iron, Zinc, and Other Trace Minerals from Vegetarian Diets. *American Journal of Clinical Nutrition* 78 (2003): 6335–6395.

Jung, A. D. Gastroesophageal Reflux in Infants and Children. *American Family Physician* 64, 11 (2001): 1853–1860.

Killip, S., J. M. Bennett, and M. D. Chambers. Iron Deficiency Anemia. *American Family Physician* 75 (2007): 671–678.

Luma, G. B., and R. T. Spiotta. Hypertension in Children and Adolescents. *American Family Physician* 73 (2006): 1158–1168.

Mellies, C. M. Is Asthma Prevention Possible with Dietary Manipulation? *Medical Journal of Australia* 177, 6 (2003): S78–S80.

Norris, J. Risk of Celiac Disease Autoimmunity and Timing of Gluten Introduction in the Diet of Infants at Increased Risk of Disease. *Journal of American Medical Association* 293, 19 (2005): 2343–2351.

Roberts, D. M., M. Ostapchuk, and J. G. O'Brien. Infantile Colic. *American Family Physician* 70 (2004): 735–740, 741–742.

Simasek, M., and D. Blandino. Treatment of the Common Cold. *American Family Physician* 75 (2007): 515–520, 522.

Index

algae-based supplements, 22
allergies, 13, 30, 32, 117, 223, 225
  first year, 13–14, 17–18
  milk, 18, 24–25, 229
  reducing risk of, 17–18
alpha-linolenic acid (ALA), 21
American Academy of Pediatrics (AAP),
    6, 199, 213
  Pediatric Nutrition Handbook, 208
American Journal of Nutrition, 3, 222
amino acids, 31
anemia, iron-deficiency, 27, 232–33
antibiotics, 188
anxiety, feeding, 29–30
appetite, 45
appetizers, 137–39
  Eggplant Caviar, 138–39
  Guacamole, 139
  Hummus, 138
apples, 59–60, 117, 191
  Apple Crisp, 172
  Apple and Pear Puree, 120–21
  Baked Apples, 172
  buying and preparation, 59–60
apricots, 60–61
  buying and preparation, 60–61
  Carrot and Apricot Puree, 120
arachidonic acid (ARA), 26, 217

artificial colors and preservatives,
  186
artificial sweeteners, 42, 182
asparagus, 61–62
  buying and preparation, 61–62
asthma, prevention of, 223
avocado, 62
  Avocado and Peach Puree, 121
  buying and preparation, 62
  Guacamole, 139
  Yogurt Avocado Dip, 140

baby. *See* first year
Baby Refried Beans, 127
Baby Safe Feeder, 38
Baby's First Beef Stew, 130
babysitters, 201
Baked Apples, 172
Baked Chicken, 167
Baked Fish, 164–65
baking, one-bowl, 142–51
balance, importance of, 56–58
bananas, 62–63, 117
  Banana Muffins, 144
  Banana with Oatmeal, 121
  buying and preparation, 62–63
  Sweet Potato and Banana Puree,
  120

barley, 63–64, 149, 219
  buying and preparation, 63–64
  Chicken Barley Stew, 129
  Vegetable Barley Soup, 153
basic baby recipes, 118–19
Basic Pancakes, 147
batch cooking, 177
beans, 21, 31, 45, 64–65, 149, 215, 221
  Baby Refried, 127
  buying and preparation, 64–65
  dried, 64
  Green Beans and Rice Puree, 120
  green and yellow, 65, 117
  Lisa's Bean, Corn, and Zucchini Stew,
    128
  Turkey Sausage Soup with Beans and
    Greens, 155
beef, 23, 65–66
  Baby's First Beef, 118
  Baby's First Beef Stew, 130
  Beef Broth, 133
  buying and preparation, 65–66
  everyday, 157–64
  Family Beef Stew, 160–61
  Hamburger Soup, 156
  hormones in, 188
  Meatballs, 157–58
  Pot Roast, 158–60
  Stuffed Cabbage, 162
  Stuffed Peppers, 163–64
  Tacos, 162–63
beets, 66–67
  buying and preparation, 66–67
Berry Dip, Very, 141
beverages, 5–6
  for preschoolers, 208
  sweetened, 5–6, 7, 40, 208
  for toddlers, 51
bibs, 12
biscuits:
  Breakfast Biscuits, 124
  Teething Biscuit, 124–25
black beans, 64
blood sugar, 45, 219–20
blueberries, 67–68
  Blueberry Cake, 175–76
  Blueberry Muffins, 144–45
  buying and preparation, 67–68

Body Mass Index (BMI), 6
books, food, 190–91
booster seat, 208
boredom, creative power of, 200
bottles:
  bedtime, 42
  cleaning, 28
  stopping, 36, 196
bowel movement, frequency of, 227–31
boxed food, 178
BRATT diet, 230
bread, 5, 68–69, 227
  buying and preparation, 68–69
  My Mother's Bread, 150–51
  whole grain, 68, 111
Breakfast Biscuits, 124
Breakfast Porridge, Overnight, 125
breastfeeding, 5, 7, 9–10, 13, 14, 17, 20,
    21, 22, 24, 26, 28, 29–31, 35, 192,
    193, 196, 217, 220, 232
  allergies and, 17–18
  bowel movements and, 227, 229,
    230
  colic and, 226
  Down syndrome child, 19
  self-regulated, 9–10, 29, 30
  teeth and, 38
  value of, 30–31
  vegan infants, 20, 21, 22
  weight gain, 19
broccoli, 69, 221
  buying and preparation, 69
Broiled Wild-Caught Salmon, 165
broth, 69–70, 131–34
  Beef, 133
  Chicken, 131
  Fresh Vegetable, 132
  pressure cooker for, 133–34
  Second Harvest Stock, 132–33
Brussels sprouts, 47, 70
  buying and preparation, 70
buckwheat, 70–71, 149
  buying and preparation, 70–71
bulgur, 71
burping, 226
butter, 24
buttermilk, 88
  muffins and pancakes, 146

cabbage, 71
  buying and preparation, 71
  Stuffed Cabbage, 161–62
caffeine, 230
cake:
  Blueberry, 175–76
  Pumpkin, 175
calcium, 6, 7, 18, 22, 25, 220–21, 222, 233
  food sources, 25, 221
  how to find superior foods with, 54
  recommended intake, 220
  for toddler, 40, 220–21
calories, 4, 210, 218
Calzone, 151–52
cancer, 26, 30, 41, 189, 215, 222
candy, 6
canned food, 178
canola oil, 76–77
car, eating in, 42
carbohydrates, 182
carrots, 72, 113, 117, 191, 236
  buying and preparation, 72
  Carrot and Apricot Puree, 120
  Carrot Pineapple Muffins, 145–46
cauliflower, 72–73
  buying and preparation, 72–73
celebratory vs. everyday eating, 213
celery, 73, 191
  buying and preparation, 73
celiac disease, 218–19
cereal, 5, 40
  infant, 11, 13, 14, 17, 30, 35, 116, 117,
    233
Certified Humane food, 188–89
cheese, 21, 24, 73–74, 221, 227
  buying and preparation, 73–74
  crackers and, 142
  Macaroni and Cheese, 168–69
  Polenta with Cheese and Roasted
    Vegetables, 170
  Yogurt Cheese Dip, 141
cherries, 74–75, 191
  buying and preparation, 74–75
  Cherri Clafouti, 173
chewing, 36, 37, 38, 42, 235
chicken, 21, 31, 75
  Baby's First Chicken, 119
  Baked Chicken, 167

  buying and preparation, 75
  Chicken Barley Stew, 129
  Chicken Broth, 131
  Chicken and Noodles, 123–24
  Chicken and Rice, 123
  Chicken and Rice Soup, 153
  Creamed Chicken, 130
  everyday, 166–67
  Roast Chicken, 166–67
chickpeas, 64
  Chickpea, Lentil, and Rice Soup,
    154
  Hummus, 138
  Lisa's Veggie and Chickpea Stew,
    127–28
childproofing, 33
Chili, Quick-Cooking, 155–56
choking, 50, 224–25
  avoiding risk of, 224–25
cholesterol, 222
chronic nonspecific diarrhea, 230–31
clementine, 75–76
colic, 32, 225–27
  dairy products and, 225–27
commercial baby food, 28, 58, 113
computer, 50
confusing issues, 214–36
consistency of food, 134
constipation, 24, 227–29, 234
  iron and, 32
  preventing, 228–29
  treating, 228
Cooke, Lucy, 48
Cookies, Oatmeal, 176–77
corn, 77–78, 149
  buying and preparation, 77–78
  Corn Muffins, 146
  Lisa's Bean, Corn, and Zucchini Stew,
    128
cornmeal (polenta), 78
  buying and preparation, 78
  Polenta with Cheese and Roasted
    Vegetables, 170
cost of food, 3, 184
  controlling, 191
country-of-origin labeling (COOL),
  186
couscous, 79

cow's milk, 17, 18, 21, 24–25, 88, 117, 196, 197, 220, 223, 229, 233
  lactose intolerance, 24–25, 229, 233–34
crackers and cheese, 142
cranberries, 79
Creamed Chicken, 130
Crohn's disease, 30
crying, in first year, 10
cucumbers, 79–80
  buying and preparation, 79–80
cupboards, childproofing, 33
cups, 12, 36, 37, 42, 196, 208

dairy products, 17, 21, 22, 45, 209
  allergies, 17, 18
  colic and, 225–27
  early childhood recommendations, 220–21
  low-fat, 215, 221
Davis, Clara, 53–54
day care, 201
dehydration, 229–30, 235
dessert, 5, 6, 7, 39, 56, 134, 195, 220
  Apple Crisp, 172
  Baked Apples, 172
  Blueberry Cake, 175–76
  Cherri Clafouti, 173
  everyday, 171–77
  Free-Form Fruit Tart, 174
  Fruit Cobbler, 172–73
  Oatmeal Cookies, 176–77
  Poached Fruit, 171–72
  Pumpkin Cake, 175
diabetes, 7, 30, 41, 189, 215, 219–20
  preventing, 219–20
  Type 1, 220
  Type 2, 219–20
diapers, 13
  changing, 29
diarrhea, 13, 25, 32, 229–31, 234
  chronic nonspecific, 230–31
  treating, 229–31
diet principles, adult, 46
dip, 140–41
  Peanut Butter, 141
  Very Berry, 141
  Yogurt Avocado, 140
  Yogurt Cheese, 141

disease, 7, 30, 215
  diet-related, 7, 41, 189–90
  prevention, 215, 218–23
diversity, 44
docosahexaenoic acid (DHA), 21–22, 26, 82, 217
  early childhood recommendations, 217
Down syndrome, 19–20
  feeding infant with, 19–20
drooling, 38–39
dry goods, 179
Dumplings, 161

edamame, 103, 104
eggplant, 80
  buying and preparation, 80
  Eggplant Caviar, 138–39
eggs, 17, 18, 21, 22, 80–81, 117, 223
  buying and preparation, 80–81
  cholesterol and, 222
  Scrambles, 122
emergency numbers, 34
encopresis, 229
enzymes, 25
equipment:
  kitchen basics, 116
  pureeing, 114–15
  safe, 33
  for starting solid foods, 12
esophagus, 232
exercise, 199–200, 229

Family Beef Stew, 160–61
family table, 50–51, 136–83, 196, 197, 198
  appetizers, 137–39
  creating a pleasant family meal, 204–205
  everyday beef, lamb, and pork, 157–64
  everyday dessert, 171–77
  everyday fish, 164–66
  everyday lunch, 151–52
  everyday poultry, 166–68
  everyday soup, 153–56
  everyday vegetarian meals, 168–71
  fruit and vegetables for dipping, 140–41
  one-bowl baking, 142–51
  power of family meal, 203–204

fast food, 4
fats, 4, 8, 40, 41, 44, 45, 53, 179, 185, 210, 215, 217, 222
    early childhood recommendations, 216–17
    for preschoolers, 210, 212
    for toddlers, 40, 41
    types of, 76–77
fatty acids, 21–22, 26, 217, 223
Feeding Infants and Toddler Study (FITS), 5–6, 40
fever, 234
    diet during, 231
fiber, 44, 45, 50, 53, 210, 222, 233, 234
    constipation and, 228, 229
    early childhood recommendations, 216
figs, 81–82
    buying and preparation, 81–82
first foods, 13–14, 30, 116–17
first year, 9–35
    basic recipes, 117–19
    breastfeeding, 5, 7, 9–10, 13, 14, 17, 20, 21, 22, 24, 26, 28, 29–31, 35, 192, 193, 196, 217, 220, 232
    crying, 10
    Down syndrome and feeding, 19–20
    fatty acids, 21–22, 26
    feeding anxiety, 29–30
    feeding guide, 14–17
    feeding schedule, 29
    first foods, 13–14, 30, 116–17
    fluoride, 27–28
    food poisoning and food-borne illnesses, 28, 114
    formula, 5, 9, 10, 11, 13, 14, 17, 20, 21, 22, 24, 26, 28, 29–30, 192, 193, 232–33
    growth in, 18–19, 30
    habits to put in place, 195
    homemade food, 117–26
    iron, 26–27, 32, 35
    lactose intolerance, 24–25, 233–34
    portion size, 18, 29
    positive feeding environment, 28–29
    preterm infant nutrition, 20
    protein needs, 21, 22, 31–32
    purees and mashed mix-ins, 119–22

raising a healthy eater, 192–95
readiness for solid food, 10–11, 13–14, 29, 30, 193
self-feeding, 17, 28, 37
self-regulation, 9–10, 12, 29, 30, 192, 194
special situations, 19–24
successful first solid meal, 14
vegetarian diets, 20–24
vitamins, 26–27, 34
water, 13
zinc, 23–24
fish, 17, 21, 31, 47, 82–84, 117, 209, 215, 217, 223
    Baby's First Fish, 119
    Baked, 164–65
    Broiled Wild-Caught Salmon, 165
    buying and preparation, 82–84
    contaminants, 82–83
    everyday, 164–66
    Fish with Pasta, 165–66
    Twice Baked Creamed Fish, 130–31
flaxseed, 84
flour substitutions, 148
fluoride, 23, 27–28
Food and Drug Administration (FDA), 187
food-borne illness, 28, 114
food industry, 3–4
    advertising, 4, 196, 197
food poisoning, 28, 187
Food Quality Protection Act (FQPA), 186
formula, 5, 9, 10, 11, 13, 14, 17, 20, 21, 22, 24, 26, 28, 29–30, 192, 193, 232–33
    bowel movements and, 227, 229, 230
    choice of, 32
    for Down syndrome child, 19
    iron in, 32, 35, 233
    lactose-free, 234
    preparation, 59
    soy, 18, 32, 104, 225
    weight gain, 19
For the Love of Food, 190
Free-Form Fruit Tart, 174
freezing baby food, 115–16, 117
french fries, 5, 6, 39, 41, 46, 117

fresh foods, 180
Fresh Vegetable Broth, 132
fruits, 3, 5, 6, 7, 21, 34, 39, 40, 45, 46, 47,
      56, 117, 189–90, 191, 198, 209, 213,
      215, 222, 228, 234
   Basic Baby Fruit Recipe, 118
   citrus, 34
   for dipping, 140
   Free-Form Fruit Tart, 174
   Fresh Fruit Salad, 122
   Fruit Cobbler, 172–73
   how to find superior foods with, 55
   juice, 6, 13, 17, 34, 40, 51, 193, 194,
      198, 208, 230, 231, 235
   organic, 59, 74, 85, 94, 95, 106, 191
   Poached Fruit, 171–72
   sugar content, 182
   for toddlers, 50, 51
   washing, 113–14
   See also specific fruits
fullness. See satiety

gas, 25, 32, 225, 226, 234
gastroesophageal reflux (GER), 24, 232
gastroesophageal reflux disease (GERD),
      232
gates, safety, 33
genetically modified (GM) foods, 187
genetics, 19, 48
Gerber Products Company, 5
germs, 28, 113–14
ginger ale, 231
gluten, and celiac disease, 218–19
gluten-free baking and cooking, 148–49,
      219
goat's milk, 24, 88
grains, 3, 5, 31, 45, 209, 210, 215
   gluten-free, 148–49
   See also whole grains
grapefruit, 84
   buying and preparation, 84
grapes, 85, 191
   buying and preparation, 85
Greens, Turkey Sausage Soup with
      Beans and, 155
growth:
   charts, 19
   first year, 18–19, 30

   preschooler, 207
   toddler, 36
growth hormone, 188
Guacamole, 139

ham, 99
Hamburger Soup, 156
heart disease, 7, 41, 215, 219, 222
height, in first year, 18–19
herbal tea, 226
high blood pressure, 7, 41, 189, 219,
      221
   preventing, 221
high chair, 12, 14, 50
   cuisine, 113–35
high-fructose corn syrup, 3, 180–81
homemade food, 113–35
   baby purees and mashed mix-ins,
      119–22
   basic recipes, 117–19
   broth, 131–34
   first foods, 116–17
   first year, 117–26
   freezing, 115–16
   pureeing, 114–15
   straining, 115
   for toddlers, 122–31
honey, 182
hormones, 45
   growth, in food, 188
hot dogs, 42
Hummus, 138
hunger, 7–8, 45
   first year, 11–12, 29
   toddler, 43, 44

illness, 7, 8
Imagination Soup, 129
independence, 43
infant feeding guide, 14–17
inferior foods, 44, 53
   avoiding, 53–54
   sodium content in, 57–58
insulin, 219, 220
iron, 11, 13, 17, 22, 24, 30, 32, 39, 53, 54,
      222
   anemia and, 27, 232–33
   in formula, 32, 35, 233

sources of, 35, 233
supplements, 26–27
irradiated food, 184, 187–88

jar food, 28, 113, 114, 178
Journal of the American Dietetic Association, 17
juice, 6, 13, 17, 34, 51, 193, 194, 198, 208, 230, 231, 235
  first year, 13
junk food, organic, 58

kidney beans, 64
kindergarten, 199
kitchen:
  clean, 28
  equipment basics, 116
  well-stocked, 177–80
kiwifruit, 85–86
  buying and preparation, 85–86
Kraft Foods, 4

lactose intolerance, 24–25, 229, 233–34
lamb, 86
  buying and preparation, 86
  everyday, 157–64
  Mediterranean Lamb Stew, 158
language, power of, 205–206
Lasagna, Lazy Vegetable, 169–70
leeks, 86–87
  Leek Soup, 154–55
lemon water, 121
lentils:
  Chickpea, Lentil, and Rice Soup, 154
  Lentil Stew, 125–26
Lisa's Bean, Corn, and Zucchini Stew, 128
Lisa's Veggie and Chickpea Stew, 127–28
local food, 186
lunch, everyday, 151–52
Lunchables, 4

macaroni and cheese, 44, 46, 50
  recipe for, 168–69
magazines, food, 137
magnesium, 222
mango, 87
  buying and preparation, 87

manners, 195, 204
mashed mix-ins, 119–22
meat, 5, 21, 31, 45, 117, 209
  Basic Baby Meat Recipe, 118–19
  everyday, 157–64
  hormones in, 188
  organic, 185
  undercooked, 114
  zinc and, 23
  See also beef; chicken; lamb; pork; turkey
Meatballs, 157–58
Mediterranean Lamb Stew, 158
Megan's Tofu Spinach Pasta Sauce, 123
melon, 87–88
  buying and preparation, 87–88
microwave, 4, 59
milk, 6, 54, 88–89, 209
  allergies, 18, 24–25, 229
  breast, 5, 7, 9–10, 13, 14, 17, 20, 21, 22, 24, 26, 28, 29, 30–31, 35, 192, 193, 196, 217, 220, 232
  buying and preparation, 88–89
  calcium content, 221
  cow's, 17, 18, 21, 24–25, 88, 117, 196, 197, 220, 223, 229, 233
  goat's, 24, 88
  lactose intolerance, 24–25, 229, 233–34
  organic, 188
  rice, 21, 89
  soy, 21, 89
  for toddler, 40, 42, 51
  types of, 88–89
  unpasteurized, 42, 114
  vitamin D in, 26
millet, 89–90, 149
  buying and preparation, 89–90
mother's group, 202
muffins, 142–46
  Banana, 144
  Blueberry, 144–45
  Buttermilk or Sour Milk, 146
  Carrot Pineapple, 145–46
  Corn, 146
  Simple, 143
  Whole-Grain, 145
  Zucchini, 143

mushrooms, 90
  buying and preparation, 90
My Mother's Bread, 150–51

naps, 29
nausea, 25, 234
navy beans, 64
nitrate poisoning, 235–36
Noodles, Chicken and, 123–24
nut butter, 21
Nutrition Action Healthletter, 3
nuts and seeds, 17, 21, 31, 90–91, 149,
    215, 222
  allergies, 17, 18
  buying and preparation, 90–91
  tree, 17, 18

oatmeal, 91
  Banana with, 121
  buying and preparation, 91
  Oatmeal Cookies, 176–77
oats, 149
obesity, adult, 6, 7, 44, 50, 189
obesity, childhood, 4, 6, 30, 41, 189, 190,
    215, 218, 219
  asthma and, 223
  preventing, 44–46, 218
  worrying about, 218
oils, 21, 40, 76–77, 179, 210, 216, 217,
    222
  types of, 76–77
olive oil, 76
omega-3 fatty acids, 21–22, 76, 82, 223
one-bowl baking, 142–51
onions, 92
  buying and preparation, 90
oral rehydration solution (ORS), 230,
    231, 235
oranges, 92–93
  buying and preparation, 92–93
organic foods, 3, 59, 114, 184, 187,
    188
  cost, 191
  junk, 58
  labeling, 59, 185
  shopping for, 185–86, 191
  terminology, 185

palmar grasp, 14
pancakes, 147–50
  Basic, 147
  Buttermilk or Sour Milk, 146
  Topping, 150
papaya, 93
  buying and preparation, 93
parchment paper, 174
parents:
  disease prevention and, 189–90
  eating advice for harried parents, 181
  effective, 202–206
  family meal and, 203–205
  food worries about toddlers, 39–42
  how good parents go bad, 42–44
  how to raise a healthy eater, 192–201
  perfect, 202–203
  power of language, 205–206
parsnips, 93–94
  buying and preparation, 93–94
pasta, 94, 227
  Fish with, 165–66
  Lazy Vegetable Lasagna, 169–70
  Macaroni and Cheese, 168–69
  Megan's Tofu Spinach Pasta Sauce,
    123
peaches, 94–95, 191
  Avocado and Peach Puree, 121
  buying and preparation, 94–95
peanuts, 17, 95
  allergies, 17, 18
  Peanut Butter Dip, 141
pears, 95, 191
  Apple and Pear Puree, 120–21
  buying and preparation, 95
  Pear and Potato Puree, 122
peas, 95–96, 117
  buying and preparation, 95–96
pediatrician, 19, 43, 44, 53, 228, 231
  choice of, 214
Pediatrics, 225
peppers, 96–97, 191
  buying and preparation, 96–97
  Stuffed Peppers, 163–64
persimmons, 97
pesticides, 185–86, 191
physical activity, 199–200, 229

phytic acid, 222
picky eaters, 6–7, 206
   coping with, 46–48
   influencing, 48
   toddlers, 46–48
pincer grasp, 14, 17
pineapple, 97–98
   buying and preparation, 97–98
   Carrot Pineapple Muffins, 145–46
pizza, 46, 183, 196, 218
plums, 98–99
   buying and preparation, 98–99
Poached Fruit, 171–72
poison control, 34
polenta. *See* cornmeal (polenta)
pollution, 223
pork, 99
   buying and preparation, 99
   everyday, 157–64
   Pork Tenderloin, 160
Porridge, Overnight Breakfast, 125
portion size, in first year, 18, 29
potassium, 53, 58
potatoes, 5, 41, 52, 99–100, 117, 191
   buying and preparation, 99–100
   Pear and Potato Puree, 122
Pot Roast, 158–60
poultry. *See* chicken; turkey
pregnancy, 17, 221, 223
preparation, food, 52, 59–112. *See also*
   specific foods
preschoolers, 198–99, 207–213
   feeding, 207–213
   four- to six-year-olds, 209–210
   growth, 207
   raising a healthy eater, 198–99
   sample meal plans, 210–13
   snacks, 210–13
   two- and three-year-olds, 209
pressure cooker, using a, 133–34
preterm infant nutrition, 20
protein, 20, 21, 45, 64, 191, 222
   animal vs. plant, 31
   in first year, 21, 22, 31–32
   how to find superior foods with, 55
   for preschoolers, 210
   sources of, 31–32

   for toddler, 40
   in vegan diet, 21, 22
Prune Sauce, Yogurt with, 126
Pudding, Vegetable, 126
Pumpkin Cake, 175
pureeing food, 114–15, 119–22

Quesadilla with Vegetables, 151
Quick-Cooking Chili, 155–56
Quick Tomato Sauce, 169
quinoa, 100–101, 149
   buying and preparation, 100–101

radishes, 101
   buying and preparation, 101
raising a healthy eater, 192–201
   first year, 192–95
   physical activity, 199–200
   preschooler, 198–99
   toddler, 196–98
raisins, 101
rapeseed oil, 76–77
rash, teething, 38–39
raspberries, 102
   buying and preparation, 102
rbST, 188
reflux, 24, 232
Refried Beans, Baby, 127
restaurants, 4, 218
rhubarb, 102
rice, 102–103, 149
   buying and preparation, 102–103
   Chicken and Rice, 123
   Chicken and Rice Soup, 153
   Chickpea, Lentil, and Rice Soup,
      154
   Green Beans and Rice Puree, 120
   milk, 21, 89
Roast Chicken, 166–67
rules, setting, 204–205
rye, 149, 219

safety, 33–34
   childproofing, 33
   equipment, 33
   food, 28, 113–14
   window, 33

salmon, 82, 83
   Broiled Wild-Caught, 165
salmonella, 80, 81
salt, 4, 6, 7, 44, 45, 53, 135, 137, 196, 221
   balance, 57–58
   in inferior foods, 57–58
   tooth, 135
sandwich ideas, 152
satiety, 8, 45, 190
   first year, 9–10, 11–12, 29
   toddler, 45
sea salt, 57
seasonings, 179
second year. *See* toddlers
scarcity model, 43
self-feeding, 17, 28, 37
   common skills, 37
self-regulation, 53
   first year, 9–10, 12, 29, 30, 192, 194
   toddler, 36, 37
shellfish, 17, 82, 83
shopping, food, 52, 59, 178, 184–91
   artificial colors and preservatives, 186
   Certified Humane food, 188–89
   controlling costs, 191
   country-of-origin labeling, 186
   genetically modified foods, 187
   growth hormone, 188
   how to, 184–91
   irradiated food, 187–88
   local food, 186
   organic food, 185–86
   for well-stocked kitchen, 177–80
shrimp, 82, 83
simethicone, 225
Simple Muffins, 143
sitting up, 13
skin cancer, 26
sleep:
   first year, 29
   preschooler, 208
   schedule, 29
smoke detectors, 33
snacks, 3, 4, 40, 44, 46, 56, 196, 218
   for preschoolers, 210–13
   salty, 6, 7
   toddler, 49–50, 196, 197
soda, 4, 5, 39

sodium, 196, 221
   high blood pressure and, 221
   in inferior foods, 57–58
   See also salt
solid foods, 5, 8, 9, 10–11, 193, 228, 236
   for Down's syndrome child, 20
   equipment needed to start feeding, 12
   favorite, 117
   foods to feed first, 13–14, 30, 116–17
   germ contamination, 28
   readiness for, in first year, 9–10, 13–14,
      29, 30, 193
   successful first meal, 14
sorbitol, 230, 231
soup, 153–56
   Chicken and Rice, 153
   Chickpea, Lentil, and Rice, 154
   everyday, 153–56
   Hamburger, 156
   Imagination, 129
   Leek, 154–55
   Quick-Cooking Chili, 155–56
   Turkey Sausage Soup with Beans and
      Greens, 155
   Vegetable Barley, 153
sour milk muffins and pancakes, 146
soy, 103–104
   allergy, 18, 225
   formula, 18, 32, 104, 225
   milk, 21, 89
   phytic acid and, 222
   tofu and tempeh, 107
soybeans, 103–104
   buying and preparation, 103–104
spinach, 104–105, 191
   buying and preparation, 104–105
   Megan's Tofu Spinach Pasta Sauce,
      123
spoon, 36, 208
   first year, 12, 14, 37, 193
squash, 105–106
steaming, 59
stew:
   Baby's First Beef, 130
   Chicken Barley, 129
   Family Beef, 160–61
   Lentil, 125–26
   Lisa's Bean, Corn, and Zucchini, 128

Lisa's Veggie and Chickpea, 127–28
Mediterranean Lamb, 158
stewing, 59
Stock, Second Harvest, 132–33
stomach, 232
ache, 234–35
acid, 28
first year, 18–19, 28
toddler, 49
stove, 33
straining food, 115
strawberries, 106, 117, 191
buying and preparation, 106
stress, 234, 235
Stuffed Cabbage, 161–62
Stuffed Peppers, 163–64
sudden infant death syndrome
(SIDS), 30
sugar, 4, 44, 45, 53, 134, 180, 195, 219–20,
224
brown, 182
cooking with, 182
excessive, for preschoolers, 211–12
in fruit, 182
how to find superior foods with,
55–56
sunlight, 26
superior foods, 44, 52–113
balance and, 56–58
guide, 59–112
how to find, 54–56
sweet potato, 106–107, 117
buying and preparation, 106–107
Sweet Potato and Banana Puree, 120
sweet tooth, 134

table food. See family table
Tacos, 162–63
tannins, 233
Tart, Free-Form Fruit, 174
teeth, 38
brushing, 224
cavities, 224
first year, 38, 224
fluoride and, 27–28
toddlers, 38–39
teething, 38–39, 229
Biscuit, 124–25

foods, 38–39
medication, 38, 42, 225
television, 50, 197, 198, 209
protecting children from, 200–201
tempeh, 21, 103, 107
buying and preparation, 107
thermometer, 231
toddlers, 36–51
beverages for, 51
designated eating location, 50–51
food worries of parents, 39–42
fruits and vegetables, 50
growth, 36
homemade food for, 122–31
how good parents go bad, 42–44
meal schedule, 36–37, 46, 49
physical activity, 199–200
picky eaters, 46–48
preventing obesity in, 44–46
raising a healthy eater, 196–98
sample menu for, 41–42
self-feeding, 37
self-regulation, 36, 37
serving two or three items, 49–50
traveling food for, 51
what to feed after twelve months, 40
tofu, 21, 103, 107, 221
buying and preparation, 107
Megan's Tofu Spinach Pasta Sauce,
123
toilet training, 228
tomatoes, 107–108
buying and preparation, 107–108
Quick Tomato Sauce, 169
toxins, 7
trans fats, 77
traveling foods, 51
tuna, 82
turkey, 23, 108–109
buying and preparation, 108–109
Turkey and Rice Soup, 153
Turkey Sausage Soup with Beans and
Greens, 155
turnip, 109
buying and preparation, 109
Twice Baked Creamed Fish, 130–31

U.S. Department of Agriculture, 185

variety, food, 44, 47, 48, 136, 194, 197
vegetables, 3, 5, 6, 7, 21, 34, 39, 40, 45,
    46, 47, 48, 56, 117, 189–90, 191, 198,
    209, 213, 215, 222, 228, 234
  Basic Baby Vegetable Recipe, 118
  cooking, 171
  for dipping, 140
  Fresh Vegetable Broth, 132
  how to find superior foods with, 55
  Lazy Vegetable Lasagna, 169–70
  Lisa's Veggie and Chickpea Stew,
    127
  nitrate levels, 236
  organic, 59, 72, 73, 96, 99, 104, 191
  Polenta with Cheese and Roasted
    Vegetables, 170
  Quesadilla with, 151
  for toddlers, 50
  Vegetable Barley Soup, 153
  Vegetable Pudding, 126
  See also specific vegetables
vegetarian diets, 20–21
  everyday meals, 168–71
  in first year, 20–24
vitamins and minerals, 18, 50
  A, 53
  B, 13, 21, 22, 23
  calcium, 6, 7, 18, 22, 25, 220–21, 222,
    233
  C, 34–35, 53, 233
  D, 11, 2, 26
  in first year, 26–27, 34
  K, 22
  superior food guide, 59–112
  supplements, 26–27
  zinc, 23–24
vomiting, 231, 234, 235
  treating, 235

water, 13, 45, 109–10, 196, 198, 208
  fluoridated, 27–28
  nitrate-contaminated, 236
  as superior food, 109–10
weight:
  birth, 18
  first year, 13, 18–19
  low birth weight, 20
  overweight, see obesity, childhood
wheat, 117, 149, 219
  allergies, 18
white food, 227
whole grains, 3, 53, 54, 56, 109–10, 137,
    196, 209, 210, 215, 222, 228, 234
  bread, 68, 111
  buying, 157
  flour, 148
  how to find superior foods with, 55
  phytic acid and, 222
  as superior food, 110–11
  Whole-Grain Muffins, 145
window safety, 33

yogurt, 21, 25, 221, 223
  buying and preparation, 111
  Yogurt Avocado Dip, 140
  Yogurt Cheese Dip, 141
  Yogurt with Prune Sauce, 126

zinc, 11, 21, 22, 39, 53, 54, 222
  in first year, 23–24
  meat and, 23
  sources of, 23–24
zucchini, 111–12
  buying and preparation, 111–12
  Lisa's Bean, Corn, and Zucchini Stew,
    128
  Zucchini Muffins, 143–44

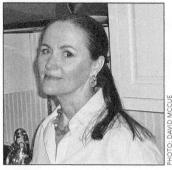

EILEEN BEHAN is a member of the American Dietetic Association (ADA) and a registered dietitian. She has twenty-five years of experience working with individuals and families. Eileen trained as a dietitian at the Brigham and Women's Hospital in Boston and completed the ADA weight-management program training for children, adolescents, and adults. She has worked for the Veterans Administration in Boston, the Harvard School of Public Health, and Seacoast Family Practice in Exeter, New Hampshire. Behan has published seven books, including the bestselling *Eat Well, Lose Weight, While Breastfeeding.* Her other books include *Microwave Cooking for Your Baby and Child; The Pregnancy Diet; Meals That Heal for Babies, Toddlers, and Children; Cooking Well for the Unwell; Fit Kids;* and *Therapeutic Nutrition.* She has written for *The Washington Post, Newsweek, Parents* magazine, *Parenting,* and *Tufts University Nutrition Newsletter.* She is a frequent lecturer on family nutrition and has been a contributor to the respected online health resource WebMD. Behan has appeared on numerous television networks and programs to discuss nutrition, including CNN, CNBC, and the *Today* show. She was the producer of *Food for Talk* on Boston public radio. She lives on the New Hampshire coast with her husband and two children.

www.eileenbehan.com